AF135002

IMMUNOLOGY AND IMMUNE SYSTEM DISORDERS

AUTOIMMUNITY VERSUS CARCINOGENESIS IN TISSUE INJURY

Immunology and Immune System Disorders

Additional books and e-books in this series can be found on Nova's website under the Series tab.

IMMUNOLOGY AND IMMUNE SYSTEM DISORDERS

AUTOIMMUNITY VERSUS CARCINOGENESIS IN TISSUE INJURY

LAWRENCE M. AGIUS

nova
Medicine & Health
New York

Copyright © 2021 by Nova Science Publishers, Inc.

All rights reserved. No part of this book may be reproduced, stored in a retrieval system or transmitted in any form or by any means: electronic, electrostatic, magnetic, tape, mechanical photocopying, recording or otherwise without the written permission of the Publisher.

We have partnered with Copyright Clearance Center to make it easy for you to obtain permissions to reuse content from this publication. Simply navigate to this publication's page on Nova's website and locate the "Get Permission" button below the title description. This button is linked directly to the title's permission page on copyright.com. Alternatively, you can visit copyright.com and search by title, ISBN, or ISSN.

For further questions about using the service on copyright.com, please contact:
Copyright Clearance Center
Phone: +1-(978) 750-8400 Fax: +1-(978) 750-4470 E-mail: info@copyright.com.

NOTICE TO THE READER

The Publisher has taken reasonable care in the preparation of this book, but makes no expressed or implied warranty of any kind and assumes no responsibility for any errors or omissions. No liability is assumed for incidental or consequential damages in connection with or arising out of information contained in this book. The Publisher shall not be liable for any special, consequential, or exemplary damages resulting, in whole or in part, from the readers' use of, or reliance upon, this material. Any parts of this book based on government reports are so indicated and copyright is claimed for those parts to the extent applicable to compilations of such works.

Independent verification should be sought for any data, advice or recommendations contained in this book. In addition, no responsibility is assumed by the Publisher for any injury and/or damage to persons or property arising from any methods, products, instructions, ideas or otherwise contained in this publication.

This publication is designed to provide accurate and authoritative information with regard to the subject matter covered herein. It is sold with the clear understanding that the Publisher is not engaged in rendering legal or any other professional services. If legal or any other expert assistance is required, the services of a competent person should be sought. FROM A DECLARATION OF PARTICIPANTS JOINTLY ADOPTED BY A COMMITTEE OF THE AMERICAN BAR ASSOCIATION AND A COMMITTEE OF PUBLISHERS.

Additional color graphics may be available in the e-book version of this book.

Library of Congress Cataloging-in-Publication Data

ISBN: 978-1-53619-610-8

Published by Nova Science Publishers, Inc. † New York

CONTENTS

PREFACE

This book is a critical appraisal of the data and evidence available in the literature of the relative roles of the immune response to neoplastic cells.

An attempt has been made to render a better understanding of the various modes of impact of the immune response against tumors in general, particularly gliomas in some of the chapters.

Autoimmune response is one mode of reactivity to native component cells within the body. Neoplastic transformation, on the other hand, critically necessitated the absence of an effective immune response to the transformed tumor cells in order for the lesion to grow and metastasise.

This book is aimed to a wide readership including in particular oncologists and the various clinical and academic professionals that care for patients with cancer. It is especially meant to provide a clear exposition of known facts regarding the genesis and further development of neoplasms, and examples of some of the commoner lesions are accounted for.

Chapter 1

Predetermined Interplay of the Projected Malignant Transformation Step as Injury Non-Resolution

Abstract

Non-resolution of carcinogenesis is a paramount consideration in the systems of non-immunogenicity of tumor cells in general and as further projected by the infiltrating glioma cell within the brain parenchyma. In such terms, the performance dynamics for further progression are change attributes that bespeak of the systems of overlap and of interactivity of multiple pathways of pro-apoptosis and of anti-apoptosis as projected by mirrored system biology of cell component injury. It is within the single transformation phenomenon step in malignancy emergence that the pro-apoptosis projects the predetermination for non-resolution of cell component injury and as further determined by non-immunogenicity of the infiltrating glioma cells.

Introduction

Cell death pathways as mechanisms in the attempted control of tumorigenesis constitute a confirmation of events within embryonic and immunologic pathways of constitutive formalization as dictated by the resultant infiltrating glioma cells within the brain parenchyma. New cancer therapies may trigger tumor necrosis and an invivo method for apoptosis detection and the early treatment response would be clinically significant; taurine (1) H magnetic resonance spectroscopy signal in gliomas may be a robust apoptotic biomarker indicative of tumor necrosis [1]. In such terms, the overall balance of pro-apoptotic and anti-apoptotic pathways is significant as equilibrating systems of biologic measures in oncogenesis per se. It is further to such considerations that apoptosis and death of malignant cells are paradoxically results of attempts at the formulation of schemes for preservation of normal parenchymal survival of CNS function and structure. Comparative genomic hybridization confirms a pattern for anaplastic oligodendrogliomas as three disjunct genetically defined subgroups of oligodendroglioma [2]. SSFA2 gene mechanism of action inhibits cell proliferation and promotes apoptosis in gliomas [3].

Cell Death Pathways

The significant degrees of control of cell death pathways are incremental dimensions that bespeak for the introduction of measures in the face of multi-pathway progression in tumorigenesis. 5-aminolevulinic acid -sonodynamic therapy with high-intensity focused ultrasound may constitute tumor specific therapy for both the tumor mass and also for infiltrating glioma cells [4].

The distinctive caspase cascades and the equally effective anti-apoptosis systems participate within the realized outgoing effects of a process of malignant transformation within the verifiable dimensions for further progression of carcinogenesis. The formulation of balancing pathways provoking apoptosis are significant in terms of the process for constitutive preservation of non-injury as defined by tissue and organ homeostasis and only secondarily as cell preservation of the life span processes of cell formulas of survival. It is in such terms that the pronounced derivation of injury to cell components and DNA perpetuates the control of homeostatic mechanisms of antigenic identity of pathways for resolute survival of pathways of progression.

It is further to such identification of antigenic identity that the final resolution of initial stages of apoptosis are pathway determination as projected by ligand/receptor binding in the first instance. MicroRNAs are aberrantly expressed in various cancers and glioma and Mir-16-5 is frequently down-regulated in astrocytomas and modulates proliferation, apoptosis and response to cytotoxic therapy [5]. Cycloartenold induces anti-proliferation on Glioma U87 cells via induction of cell cycle arrest and p38 MAPK-mediated apoptosis [6]. Such terms of resolution demand a formula for progression that is conveyed paradoxically by the carcinogenesis complex of interactivities and further constitutional determination by pro-apoptotic and anti-apoptotic pathways of non-resolution.

Identifiable Parameters of Progression

Proportional identification of injury to components of a cell are identification clues to a paramount determination as conveyed by systems of progression of such cell component injury. The emergence of such realization is pathway progression of the pro-apoptosis within schemes of attempted anti-apoptosis.

The further predetermination of cell injury is within schemes of projection as determined by antigenicity, on the one hand, and of receptor confirmation of binding of such antigens as indeed determined by formulas of injury progression in cells undergoing apoptosis.

DYSHOMEOSTASIS

The complex dyshomeostasis as confirmed and further realized in cells undergoing apoptosis is pathway delineation that extensively coordinates the outcome projection of systems for progression. Long non-coding RNA plays a crucial role in the progression of glioma and promotes glycolysis by regulating miR-152-3p/SLC2A1 axis in glioma [7]. The identity constitution of pathways of non-resolution of pro-apoptotic pathways is characterization of the essential features of the malignant change that transforms normal glial cells to infiltrating glioma cells. Compound 6d (ursolic acid derivative) promotes apoptosis in glioma cells through down-regulation of cAMP [8]. Such measures within systems for progression are integral determinants of the malignant transformation as borne out by numerous cell types and within systems of essential non-resolution of cell component injury.

The apoptosis of such transforming cells is further projected as confirmatory systems predisposing to injury to DNA and to immunologic components of identification and realization. Photodynamic therapy with hematoporphyrin significantly increases cell apoptosis, induces the content of reactive oxygen species and decreases the mitochondrial membrane potential and thus indicating induced apoptosis [9]. The proportional dispersal of the injurious agent within cell component biologic mechanisms is a further determination of progression of the apoptosis that identifies and further confirms the projection of the malignant transformation process beyond ligand-receptor binding of such components as CD95 and ApoL ligands to their constitutive receptors. Gpx 4 is implicated in the proliferation, migration and apoptosis of glioma cells [10]. In terms therefore of identifiable constitution, the realization of injury to cells is itself a potent mechanistic determinant in a malignant transformation step in carcinogenic identification.

Pro-Apoptosis and Anti-Apoptosis

The significance of emergence of a balance between pro-apoptosis and anti-apoptosis is projected as system biology of multiple models for attempted resolution of a carcinogenesis within further system pathways of injury that in turn determines outcome dynamics for non-resolution of cell component injury. PSMB8 interference may inhibit the migration and proliferation of glioma cells by reducing expression of cyclin A, cyclin B1, cyclin D1, vimentin, and N-cadherin, and by increasing expression of E-cadherin through modulation of ERK2/3 and PI3K/AKT signaling pathways [11]. The performance determinants of malignant transformation are system pathways that overlap with confirmatory realization as conveyed by the progressiveness of the malignant transformation step undergone by constitutive cells. It is within the further development of mechanistic pathways of such non-resolution that the emergence of tumorigenesis is both identifiable and further projected by systems of overlap and of redundancy as afforded by pro-apoptosis.

The significant identification of non-immunogenicity is conveyed by infiltrating glioma cells within the system biology of mirrored images as geometrically determined by the overall malignant lesion extending within the brain parenchyma.

Performance Attributes

Performance attributes significantly determine the identity of non-resolution as further predetermination of the pro-apoptosis as targeted within systems of biologic progression of the infiltrating glioma cell. Fibronectin 1 exerts a potent role in stimulating glioma growth, invasion and survival through the activation of the PI3K/AKT signaling pathway [12]. The atypical protein kinase RIOK3 contributes to glioma cell proliferation/survival, migration/invasion and the AKT/mTOR signaling pathway [13]. In such terms, the outcome dynamics for non-resolution are integral to a non-immunogenicity that is identifiable determinant of injury non-resolution in its own right.

The performance hence of non-resolution as projected by progression of pro-apoptosis pathways is hence a significant contribution as portrayed within the pathways of simple predetermination as exerted by carcinogenic agents of multi-identity.

Conclusion

The delivery of both pro-apoptosis and anti-apoptosis are signal pathways of consequential import, as identifiable by modification of systems of potential malignant transformation to an infiltrating glioma cells. It is such realization that affords the identification of a malignant transformation step as attribute determination of the infiltrating glioma cells. Proportional emergence is delivery confirmation within determinant systems of exchange and interactivity as cell component injury.

The emergence of a single step in malignant transformation is identifiable within the modeled system biology of such interactivity of pathway progression and interactivity as systems of projected potent predetermination of the constitutive glioma cells. The infiltrative phenotype is characterized as significant component biology that arises within effects projected by the non-immunogenicity of the infiltrating tumor cells and as further confirmed by dynamics of non-resolution.

References

[1] Opstad KS, Bell BA, Griffiths JR, Howe FA "Taurine: a potential marker of apoptosis in gliomas" *Br J Cancer* 2009;100(5):789-94.

[2] Koschny R, Heidrun Holland H, Koschny T, Vitzthum HE "Comparative genomic hybridisation pattern of non-anaplastic and

anapaestic oligodendrogliomas—a meta-analysis" *Pathol Res Pract* 2006; 202(1):23-30.

[3] Zhu A, Li X, Wu H, Miao Z, Yuan F, Zhang F et al. "Molecular mechanism of SSFA2 deletion inhibiting cell proliferation and promoting cell apoptosis in glioma" *Pathol Res Pract* 2019;215(3): 600-606.

[4] Suehiro S, Ohnishi T, Yamashita D, Kohno S, Inoue A, Nishikawa M et al. "Enhancement of antitumor activity by using 5-ALA-mediated sonodynamic therapy to induce apoptosis in malignant gliomas: significance of high-intensity focused ultrasound on 5-ALA-SDT in a mouse glioma model" *J Neurosurg* 2018;129(6):1416-1428.

[5] Krill A, Wolter M, Stojcheva N, Hertler C, Liesenberg F, Zapata M et al. "MiR-16-5p is frequently down-regulated in astrocytic gliomas and modulates glioma cell proliferation, apoptosis an response to cytotoxic therapy" *Neuropathol Appl Neurobiol* 2019;45(5):441-458.

[6] Liu H, Li X, Yang A, Jin Z, Wang X, Wang Q et al. "Cycloartenol exerts anti-proliferative effects on Glioma U87 cells via induction of cell cycle arrest and p38 MAPK-mediated apoptosis" *J Buon* 2018;23(6):1840-1845.

[7] She J, Zhang Y, Qin B, Wang Y, Zhu X "Long non-coding RNA LINC00174 promotes glycolysis and tumor progression by regulating miR-152-3p/SLC2A1 axis in glioma" *J Exp Clin Cancer Res* 2019;38(1):395.

[8] Fan H, Geng L, Yang F, Dong X, He D, Zhang Y "Ursolic acid derivative induces apoptosis in glioma cells through down-regulation of cAMP" *Eur J Med Chem* 2019;176:61-67.

[9] Yuan SX. Li JL, Xu XK, Chen W, Chen C, Kuang KQ et al. "Underlying mechanism of the photodynamic activity of hematoporphyrin-induced apoptosis in U87 glioma cells" *Int J Mol Med* 2018;41(4): 2288-2296.

[10] Zhao H, Ji B, Chen J, Huang Q, Lu X "Gpx r is involved in the proliferation, migration and apoptosis of glioma cells" *Pathol Res Pract* 2017;213(6):626-633.

[11] Yang BY, Song JW, Sun HZ, Xing JC, Yang ZH, Wei CY et al. "PSMB8 regulates glioma cell migration, proliferation, and apoptosis through modulating ERK1/2 and PI3K/AKT signaling pathways" *boomed Pharmacother* 2018;100:205-212.

[12] Liao YX, Zhang ZP, Zhao J, Liu JP "Effects of fibronectin 1 on cell proliferation, senescence and apoptosis of human glioma cells through the PI3K/AKT signaling pathway" *Cell Physiol Biochem* 2018;48(3):1382-1396.

[13] Zhang T. Ji D, Wang P, Liang D, Jin L, Shi H et al. *The atypical protein kinase RIOK3 contributes to glioma cell proliferation/ survival, migration/invasion and the AKT/mTOR signaling pathway.*

Chapter 2

Systems of Active Immune Suppression as Integral Malignant Transformation in Infiltrating Glioma Cells

Abstract

Immunologic tolerance to an infiltrating tumor cell bed is a very active process of suppression of the immune responsive mechanisms with a strong executive process of regressive adaptation of the adjacent infiltrated brain tissues. In such terms, constitutive realization of the malignant transformation process is a derived series of homeostatic mechanisms that adaptively come to adopt the significant aberrancy of a nonresponse on the part of systems of recognition and also of execution as borne out by the appraisal process of institutionalized pathways of attempted response to the infiltrating tumor cells.

Introduction

The concentrated approach to the evolutionary development of primary malignant gliomas constitutes in reality an appreciation of events centered on cytokine production and delivery to the tumor cell bed, as primarily exemplified by resection cavity creation after subtotal surgical removal. Podoplanin-positive myeloid cells with transcriptional regulation of arginase-1 are one class of mediators of the glioma-modulated immune suppression [1]. Glioblastoma patients have a significant elevation of myeloid-derived suppressor cells in peripheral blood but not immunosuppressive Tregs [2]. The consequent delineation of injury to tumor cells is coupled to the presence of a blood brain barrier functionality and dysfunctionality. In such terms, the emergence of injury to neoplastic cells primary in the central nervous system (CNS) constitutes in itself the evolutionary hallmark of a series of immunologic attempts at potential eradication of the tumor lesion. Glioblastoma takeover involves soluble factors such as chemokine and cytokines, direct cell-cell contact, extracellular vesicles and micro-vesicles and connecting nanotubes and microtubes [3]. It is further to such concerns that the complete evolutionary nature of injury to tumor cells is beset by the delineation of a lesion that both infiltrates and proliferates in terms of a series of developmentally regressive changes.

CYTOKINES

It is significant to view cytokine delivery systems as integral to the potential antitumor responses of the immune system in terms that abrogate the host's environmental disposition to evade such immune responses. Toll-like receptor 2 enhances glioma immune evasion by down-regulating MHC Class II molecules in microglia [4]. It is within encompassed derivation of the neoplastic lesion that infiltration of the surrounding brain tissue dominates, in real terms, in the evolutionary adaptation of the CNS to a lesion that is suppressed immunologically. Activated dendritic cells, eosinophils, activated mast cells, monocytes and activated natural killer cells positively relate to prognosis of glioma patients whereas resting natural killer cell, CD8+ T cells, T follicular helper cells, gamma delta T cells and M0 macrophages negatively relate to prognosis [5]. The emergence of cell injury to a highly infiltrative and highly proliferative neoplastic lesion is beset by the spread phenomenon that diffusely compromises dynamics of turnover of immune cells within the CNS.

Blocking myeloid-derived suppressor cells holds great promise for enhancing the efficacy of gene therapy-mediated immunotherapies for glioblastoma [6].

Constitutional Factors

Constitutive dynamics of recognition of tumor-associated antigens are de facto a system of failed retrieval within the immune system turnover and of the failed constitutive amplification of the antitumor immune response. Self-renewing cancer stem cells in glioblastoma possess expression of TLR4 that permits them to survive in spite of inflammatory signals [7].

In such terms, the further definition of injury to a primary tumor cell bed is hampered by the emergence of such features as the infiltrative proliferation inherent to malignant glioma evolutionary course. It is within systems for potent infiltrative definition that the primary malignant glioma both constitutes and further informs the significant suppression of an active immune response as primary consideration in primary tumor biology.

The performance dynamics, as borne out by a system of primal infiltration, includes the delineation of an immune response that potentially can be activated in terms of antitumor potent response. In such terms, the outline phenomenon of infiltration of adjacent brain tissue is derivative process within the biologic evolution of the primary malignant glioma as relative to the proliferative biology of the glioma cells themselves.

In such terms, ongoing immune responsiveness is dynamic constitution as evolutionary substitution of normal homeostatic mechanisms as projected beyond the adjacent brain tissues. Several immunotherapies are being tested including inhibition of immune checkpoint regulators, antitumor vaccination from dendritic cell and tutor peptide components, adoptive transfer of supercharged and durable T lymphocytes, and the use of oncolytic viruses [8].

Conditioned Settings

The emerging conceptual settings of a primary neoplasm are derived dynamics of an injury that provokes proliferation of infiltrating cells in the first instance. Primarily infiltrating tumor cells are significantly dynamic in terms of resultant turnover processes of attempted renewal of the malignant transformation phenomenon. In such terms, ongoing derivative regression biologically and pathophysiologically is a failure of the responsiveness of the immune system that dynamically attempts at adaptation to altered homeostatic mechanisms. An essential turnover process lies at the heart of a concentrated effort to evade the immune responses within systems for further primary infiltrative behavior.

In such terms, ongoing redistribution of various metabolic substrates is subservient phenomenon within dynamic systems of primarily altered adaptation. It is further to such considerations that the overall homeostasis systems are adaptive to and also primarily inducive to a failed immunologic response to primarily infiltrative tumor cell beds. In addition to heterogeneous populations of tutor cells, glioma stem cells and other nontumor cells in the glioma microenvironment serve as critical regulators of tutor progression and recurrence [9]. Suppression of antitumor T cell immunity has been shown by the oncometabolite (R)-2-hydroxyglutarate [10].

Immune Response

Significant terms of attempted retrieval of the immune response to a malignant glioma is textual verification of an injury to glial cells that is portrayed and further projected as malignant transformation of a primarily infiltrating tumor cell population and of a series of further infiltrative phenomena. It is in such terms that the ongoing regression of a lesion is beset by a failure to recover an immune responsiveness within systems of dynamic turnover.

The performance attributes of such injury towards malignant transformation derive significance as terms of relative insufficiency of a primary and of a secondary immune response. It is clearly within such concept of integrative suppression of response that the derived phenomenon of re-constitutive biology both fails as homeostatic mechanism and also as derived turnover overactivity as projected in terms of performance dynamics. Missense mutations in the active site of isocitrate dehydrogenase 1 (IDH1) biologically and also diagnostically distinguish low-grade gliomas and secondary glioblastomas from primary glioblastomas; mutant isocitrate dehydrogenase 1 expression drives gliomagenesis, mutant IDH1 itself is rapidly converted from driver to passenger [11]. In addition to R(-)-2-hydroxyglutarate, alterations in several other metabolites measured by magnetic resonance spectroscopy correlate with IDH1 mutation status [12].

ABERRANT IMMUNE RESPONSE

A primary aberrant immune response accounts for repression of an immune response that is homeostatically conditioned and reconditioned within systems of adaptive pathology of systems of pathogenesis of the malignant transformation process.

There is increasing evidence that the dysregulated metabolic activity of neoplastic cells generates an immunosuppressive tutor microenvironment that orchestrates an impaired anti-timor immune response [13].

Novel combination treatments are warranted such as inhibition of histone deacetylases1/2 and of TRAP1 to induce synthetic lethality in glioblastomas [14].

In such terms, evolutionary derivation is both etiology and pathogenesis of an injury that recharacterizes the homeostatic mechanics of a proliferating tumor cell bed within systems of an aberrant immune response that in turn is responsible for the primarily infiltrative phenomenon. It is such setting that accounts for redefinition of tumor cell biology within confines of an abnormal reconditioning of a process of malignant transformation.

CONCLUSION

Dynamics of attempted reconstitution are failure dynamics of a homeostatic conditioning within contextual reappraisal of a suppressed immune response to primarily infiltrating tumor cells of a malignant glioma lesion. In such terms, the derivative phenomenon of suppressive phenomena is integral to a biology of responsiveness within systems of active recognition of tumor-associated and tumor-specific antigens.

The cooperative evolutionary performance of integral dynamics further constitutes a system of immune tolerance as dictated by an aberrant series of immune responses. Significant emphasis is being made on targeting class II MHC transcription factors to either inhibit or stimulate the immune response in, especially, cell-based vaccines [15].

It is clearly the nature of aberrant responses that permissively condition such responses to active suppression as dictated by the infiltrative process of the tumor cells. It is further to such proposed dynamics that immune tolerance is a very active process of regressive adaptation within systems of both recognition and suppression of the immune system to the real immunologic identities of the infiltrative tumor cell bed.

REFERENCES

[1] Eisemann T, Costa B, Peterziel H, Angel P "Podoplanin positive myeloid cells promote glioma development by immune suppression" *Front Oncol* 2019;9:187.

[2] Alban TJ, Alvarado AG, Sorensen MD, Bayik D, Volovetz J, Serbinowski E, Mulkearns-Hubert EE et al. "Global immune fingerprinting in glioblastoma patient peripheral blood reveals immune-suppression signatures associated with prognosis" *JCI Insight* 2018;3(21):e122264.

[3] Broekman ML, Maas SLN, Abels ER, Mempel TR, Krichevsky AM, Breakefield XO "Multidimensional communication in the micro environs of glioblastoma" *Nat Rev Neural* 2018;14(8):482-495.

[4] Qian J, Luo F, Yang J, Liu J, Liu R, Wang L et al. "TLR2 promotes glioma immune evasion by down regulating MHC Class II molecules in microglia" *Cancer Immunol Res* 2917;6(10):1220-1233.

[5] Zhong QY, Fan EX, Feng GY, Chen QY, Gou XX, Yue GJ et al. "A gene expression-based study on immune cell subtypes and glioma prognosis" *BMC Cancer* 2019;19(1):1116.

[6] Kamran N, Kadiyala P, Saxena M, Candolfi M, Li Y, Moreno-Ayala MA et al. "Immunosuppressive myeloid cells ' blockade in glioma microenvironment enhances the efficacy of immune-stimulatory gene therapy" *Mol There* 2017;25(1):232-248.

[7] Alvarado AG, Thiagarajan PS, Mulkearns-Hubert EE, Silver DJ, Hale JS, Alban TJ et al. "Glioblastoma cancer stem cells evade innate immune suppression of self-renewal through reduced TLR4 expression" *Cell Stem Cell* 2017;20(4):450-461.

[8] Wilcox JA, Ramakrishna R, Magge R "Immunotherapy in glioblastoma" *World Neurosurg* 2018;116:518-528.

[9] Ma Q, Long W, Xing C, Chu J, Luo M, Wang HY et al. "Cancer Stem cells and immunosuppressive microenvironment in glioma" *Front Immunol* 2018;9:2924.

[10] Bunse L, Pusch S, Bunse T, Sahm F, Sanghvi K, Friedrich M, et al. "Suppression of antitumor T cell immunity by the oncometabolite (R)-2-hydroxyglutarate" *Nat Med* 2018;24(8):1192-1203.

[11] Johannessen TC A, Mukherjee J, Viswanath P, Ohba S, Ronen S, Bjerkvig R et al. "Rapid conversion of mutant IDH1 from driver to passenger in a model of human gliomagenesis" *Mol Cancer Res* 2016;14(10):965-983.

[12] Pope WB, Prins RM, Thomas MA, Nagarajan R, Yen KE, Bitsiger MA et al. "Non-invasive detection of 2-hydroxyglutarate and other metabolites in IDH1 mutant glioma patients using magnetic resonance spectroscopy" *J Neurooncol* 2012;107(1):197-205.

[13] Jiang Z, Hsu JL, Li Y, Hortobagyi GN, Hung MC "Cancer cell metabolism bolsters immunotherapy resistance by promoting an immunosuppressive tumor microenvironment" *Front Oncol* 2020;10:1197.

[14] Nguyen TTT, Zhang Y, Shang E, Shu C, Quinzii CM, Westhoff MA et al. "Inhibition of HDAC1/2 along with TRAP1 causes synthetic lethality in glioblastoma model systems" *Cells* 2020;9(7):1661.

[15] Radosevich M, Ono SJ "Novel mechanisms of class II major histocompatibility complex gene regulation" *Immunol Res* 2003;27(1):85-106.

Chapter 3

SYSTEMS OF FAILURE OF IMMUNE RESPONSE TO EARLY CARCINOGENESIS RECHARACTERIZE SUCH EARLY CARCINOGENESIS

ABSTRACT

The characterization of injury to normal cells in terms of an early stage in carcinogenesis is a re-characterization of the modulated stage of emergence of a failed immune response to such early carcinogenesis. It is significant to consider modulatory steps in evolution of the neoplastic lesion in terms that beget further suppression of the immune system to survey the landscape modulatory potentials for further growth of the tumor and its often quasi concurrent mechanisms of spread within the body. It is therefore in terms of a significant concurrent series of events that formulation of the early carcinogenesis is inherently coupled to events of a suppression of the immune response as re-characterized systems of essential emergence of progressiveness.

Introduction

The conceptual approach to treat established tumors rather than to prevent tumorigenesis is a fundamental consideration within the domains of progressive evolution of given tumors that expand and grow towards the metastatic spread of the lesions. Tripartite motif (TRIM) family proteins, most of which have E3 ubiquitin ligase activities influence intracellular signaling, development, apoptosis, protein quality control, innate immunity, autophagy and carcinogenesis [1]. Such concept is further important as enveloping deterministic considerations of the presence of tumor antigens that are also often expressed by normal tissues. Alarmins are involved as initiators and participants in host defense, gene expression regulation, homeostasis, inflammation, autoimmunity and oncogenesis [2]. In such terms, the emergence of tumor lesions is a realization of a malignant transformation of initially normal tissues, but normal in relative consideration only. cGAS-STING has dichotomous roles in tumor development and immunity [3]. The evolution of normal tissues is an evolving concept in its own right, within the further relative relevance as a source for tumors that spread in differential terms. The incremental dimensions of realization of tumor growth and spread are themselves only relatively related in that inceptive neoplasms may spread at initial stages of evolution of these lesions.

Incremental Evolution

The incremental evolutionary development of tumors is a deterrent in the development of cancer vaccines that are to a significant extent a measure aimed at eradicating the tumor at a specific developmental stage of growth and spread of the lesion. Inflammation predisposes to the development of cancer and promotes all stages of tumorigenesis [4]. In such terms, the further participation of injury to actively dividing and also dynamically stationary tumor cells is a concept based only on theoretical considerations. Intestinal microbiota are linked to colorectal carcinogenesis in terms of inflammation induction, genotoxin biosynthesis interfering with cell cycle regulation, and the production of toxic metabolites [5]. The human microbiome is an emerging target in cancer development and therapeutics and is directly oncogenic through mucosal inflammation or systemic dysregulation [6]. The relative dimensions of the evolutionary character of a given tumor lesion are therefore of important import within the dynamic landscape of a mitotic lesion that continually and forcefully evades the immune system reactivities. It is significant to consider the vaccination program proposed for eradication of a given tumor lesion as a simplistic concept with regard to emergence of neo-antigens that further propel the carcinogenesis program of growth and spread of the lesion.

STAGES OF EMERGENCE

It is further to such considerations to realize that the emergence of tumors constitutes in itself a fundamental step in the evolutionary program of the immune response to act against the initial steps of carcinogenesis. Occasionally, immune-mediated elimination of human Papilloma virus infection of cervical cells fails with increased expression of the E6 and E7 oncoprotein resulting in disrupted cell cycle, cell proliferation and malignant transformation, and induced immunosuppression [7]. It is significant to realize that the immune response is at early stages of tumorigenesis a failed immune response to the cancer lesional evolution. Virally infected cells can acquire cancer hallmarks, especially after induced immunosuppression and exposure to co-carcinogenic stimuli [8]. The importance of such considerations is the direct projection of carcinogenesis as terms of reference to such early failure of the immune responses to eradicate such given tumor lesion.

The realization of an injurious insult to early transforming event in carcinogenesis is the failure to suppress the malignant transformation events at the early inceptive stage of lesion development. In such terms, emergence of carcinogenesis as a progressive evolution is tantamount realization of events that persist indefinitely within systems of modulation of the immune system.

Immune Response

The immune response is itself a biologic determinant at early stages of carcinogenesis within simple evolutionary terms of systems of biologic modification based largely on dynamic interactivities with the emerging tumor lesion. Immune evasion by tumors involves targeting the regulatory T cell function or secretions, antigen presentation, modifying production of suppressive immune mediators, tolerance and immune deviation [9]. The emergence of carcinogenesis is a consideration in terms of the failed constitutive response of the immune system in its attempts to eradicate the neoplastic lesion. Tumor immunosuppressive networks include regulatory T cells, natural killer T cells and distinct subgroups of immature and mature dendritic cells [10]. The pervasive evolutionary course of the tumor is thus a characterization of many essential facets of the failure program of an otherwise potentially responding immune system to early stages of carcinogenesis.

Developmental Waves

Developmental waves of progression of the tumor lesion are additional factors in the projection of metastatic spread in terms of evolution of the neoplasm. The full realization of a carcinogenesis is persistent during the whole evolutionary course of the lesion.

The carcinogenesis phenomenon is a fully operative basis for the progressive evolutionary course of a neoplastic lesion that gains potential for further progressive growth and spread within the body. It is significant to consider evolution as a dynamic and reactive adaptation to accommodating facets of the immune response. CD4(+)CD25(high) T regulatory cells (Treg) are important mediators of active immune evasion in cancer [11]. The emergence of such significant import further translates the immune response in terms of modulatory influences that are themselves characterizations of the intrinsic early carcinogenesis phenomenon. Some recent studies have demonstrated that myeloid-derived suppressor cell targeting improves the efficacy of immune checkpoint blockade in cancer therapy [12].

MODULATION

Such considerations are suggestive of the presence of an all pervasive and dominant phenomenon that modulates both the early carcinogenesis process and the modulated failure of the immune response such as early stages of the carcinogenetic process. In such terms, the biologic basis for the immune response is a modulated and re-characterized process of mutual suppression of both T and B lymphocytes.

Such a concept is suggestive of a suppression and dominant phenomenon within the genetic landscape dynamics of the given tumor lesion. Perforce reinterpretation of dynamics of tumor evolution is significant in terms of the essential process of emergence of the tumor lesion as concurrent failure of an immune response as re-characterized essential features of the early carcinogenesis process. This is a term of reference within simple project models of the evolutionary course of a given neoplasm as encompassed derivation of the lesion from originally normal tissues of origin of the tumor.

Tumor-related suppression mechanisms include accumulations of adenosine-reducing regulatory T-cells, release of suppressive micro-vesicles by tumor cells, and expression of toll-like receptors on the tumor cell surface [13].

Such a conceptual background for the early carcinogenesis may elucidate the nature of tumorigenesis as both progressive and persistently capable of spread within a body system of nonresponse of the immune reactivities. It is significant to recognize such a phenomenon that is inherently persistent in terms of the failures of the immune reactivities and responses in suppressing the tumorigenesis growth and spread of the given lesion.

Conclusion

The uniformity of failure dynamics of the immune response as permissive failure to suppress the tumorigenesis is a strict characterization of the lesion as fundamentally mutual evolutionary steps in carcinogenesis. The emergence step in such carcinogenesis is a strict re-characterization of immune biology in terms of the modulation of the malignant transformation step. The emergence, in turn, of conceptual redefinition of such malignant transformation is the fundamental character of progressiveness of a lesion that is potentially modulatory and re-modulatory within the evasive dimensions of the tumor lesion processes of growth and spread within immune system non surveillance dynamics. The perforce contributions of such failed immune surveillance is permissive in terms arising from dynamics of recognition and reactivity by the immune system. In terms, therefore, of overall consequence, the emergence of early stages of carcinogenesis incorporate the nature of failure of the immune response to suppress tumorigenesis as emergent process of malignant transformation of essentially normal tissues in first instance.

References

[1] Hatakeyama S "Trim family proteins: roles in autophagy, immunity, and carcinogenesis" *Trends Biochem Sci* 2017;42(4):297-311.

[2] Yang D, Han Z, Oppenheim JJ "Alarmins and immunity" *Immunol Rev* 2007;280(1):41-56.

[3] Ng KW, Marshall EA, Bell JC, Lam WL "cGAS-STING and cancer: dichotomous roles in tumor immunity and development" *Trends Immune* 2018;39(1):44-54.

[4] Greten FR, Grivennikov SI "Inflammation and cancer: triggers, mechanisms, and consequences" *Immunity* 2019;51(1):27-41.

[5] Lucas C, Barnich N, Nguyen HTT "Microbiota, inflammation and colorectal cancer" *Int J Mol Sci* 2017;18(6): 1310.

[6] Ricardo SL, Coburn B, Hansen AR "The microbiome and cancer for clinicians" *Crit Rev Oncol Hematol* 2019;141:1-12.

[7] Vonsky M, Shabaeva M, Runov A, Lebedeva N, Chowdhury S, Palesfsky JM et al. "Carcinogenesis associated with Human Papillomavirus infection. Mechanisms and potential for immunotherapy" *Biochemistry (Mosc)* 2019;84(7): 782-799.

[8] Gaglia MM, Munger K "More than just oncogenes: mechanisms of tumorigenesis by human viruses" *Curr Opin Virol* 2018;32:48-59.

[9] Vilay DS, Ryan EP, Pawelec G, Taleb WH, Stagg J, Elkord E et al. "Immune evasion in cancer: mechanistic basis and therapeutic strategies" *Semin Cancer Biol* 2015;35 Suppl:S185-198.

[10] Rabinovich GA, Gabrilovich D, Sotomayor EM "Immunosuppressive strategies that are mediated by tumor cells" *Annu Rev Immune* 2007;25:267-96.

[11] Menetrier-Caux C, Curiel T, Faget J, Manuel M, Caux C, Zou W "Targeting regulatory T cells" *Target Oncol* 2012;7(1): 15-28.

[12] Toor SM, Elkord E "Therapeutic prospects of targeting myeloid-derived suppressor cells and immune checkpoints in cancer" *Immunol Cell Biol* 2018;96(6):888-897.

[13] Whiteside TL, Mandapthil M, Szczepanski M, Szajnik M "Mechanisms of tumor escape from the immune system: adenosine-producing Treg, exosomes and timor-associated TLRs" *Bull Cancer* 2011;98(2): E25-31.

Chapter 4

MIRROR IMAGES OF GEOMETRIC PRE-SETTING OF THE INFILTRATING EDGES OF HIGH-GRADE GLIOMAS

ABSTRACT

Dimensional reproducibility of the malignant transformation step is integral to a parental tumor mass that grows largely as infiltrating edges within the adjacent brain parenchyma surrounding, in geometric fashion, the growing or recurrent high-grade glioma. In such terms, overall predetermination is genetic and constitutive biology of a repertoire of adhesion molecules that beset the realization of tumor cell injury as performance attribute of the infiltrating tumor edge. The redistributive phenomena of constitutive performance appear mirror-image projection of a glioma that infiltrates rather than grows directly as a parental mass and, as signified by, systems of projected induction of adhesion molecular biology.

INTRODUCTION

The distinction between the various specificities of adhesion molecule affinity to extra-cellular molecules includes the derivative dimensions of infiltrative and mobility phenomena within systems of evolving tumorogenesis. The mechanism of angiogenesis and invasion induce the production of an array of adhesion molecules and extracellular matrix (ECM) components [1]. An important mechanism mediating neural regulation of gliomas is activity-dependent cleavage and section of the synaptic adhesion molecule neuroligin-3 which enhances glioma proliferation through the PI3K-mTOR pathways [2]. In such terms, the overall compass of biologic intervention within gliomas and other tumor types calls into operative consideration the evolving dimensions of inclusive manipulation as inhibition of such infiltrativeness. Roles of the adhesion molecules on glia (AMOG) and L1CAM (L1) in glioma cells correlate with tumorigenesis [3]. It is within systems of manipulative induction that a whole series of arrays of substitutive mechanisms are stimulated as performance induction of physico-biologic involvement. The system array phenomenon is further cooperative dimension as portrayed by the necessity for induction that overall qualifies in terms of inclusive systems of both extracellular matrix and cell-surface molecules, on the one hand, and of receptors for the extracellular matrix and cell-surface adhesion molecules, on the other hand.

Derivative Mechanisms

Derivative inclusions of adhesion molecules as mechanisms of manipulative tools for the development of inhibition of infiltration by glioma cells are systems for portrayal phenomena that complex glioma biology with the evolving proliferation and cell genesis as systems of projection. Adhesion molecules on glioma cells, tumor-infiltrating lymphocytes, and endothelial cells within the neoplasm offer insight in the molecular basis of the interaction between glioma cells and heterologous cells types in the tumor environment and between tumor cells and the extracellular matrix [4]. The performance attributes for rearrangement and induction are applicable to adhesion molecules that preferentially localize post-surgical tumor residual to the walls of the resection tumor cavity. In such terms, the evolving surgical residual tumor bed involves the derivative dimensions, as mirrored by systems of inclusive phenomena, as applicable to adhesion molecule biology.

System Injury Profiles

The realization of injury to tumor cells is well exemplified by the use of radio-immuno conjugates that evolve within the realized schemes of projected susceptibilities of the neoplastic cells. Gliomas are participants within the performance projections of an injury that is prolonged as potential system pathways of induced vulnerability of the tumor bed.

The residual dimensions are susceptible targets as portrayed by a maximum dose-radiation field that includes essentially infiltrating edges of a partially resected glioma. Accordingly, the further conformational mirror-image dimensions are, in a real sense, the attribute derivative of a whole series of overlapping systems of induced stimulation, and as also opportune susceptibility to tumor cell injury. Cell adhesion molecule 2 inhibits human glioma tumorigenesis by modulating the cell cycle and the epithelial mesenchymal transition markers including E-cadherin and beta-catenin [5].

The performance realization of injury to transformed cells has unique as well as overlapping adhesion molecular biology attributes. In such terms, the conformational involvement of infiltrative glioma cells is integral to a redefinition of tumor biology as terms of reference to an ongoing normal or abnormal brain biology adjacent and adherent to such infiltrating glioma cells. The formation of abnormal vasculature to tumors and glioma cell invasion along white matter tracts appear to lead to resistance of gliomas to treatment [6]. It is significant to view tumor infiltration within scopes of transformed or reactive adhesion molecules in the realization of induced action, as manipulative systems of egress or inclusion. The receptor-ECM component interaction is critical to glioma cell invasion into the adjacent brain tissue involving the integrin superfamily adhesion receptors and CD44 [7, 8].

MIRROR REPRODUCIBILITY

The model of mirror reproducibility of the primal malignant transformation step is directional intervention, as borne out by systems of infiltration of the adjacent brain parenchyma. In such hierarchical terms, the dominance of infiltration by tumor cells is provocative phenomenon within encompassed realization of a series of activities determined by adhesion molecular biology. Cells stimulated by fibronection expressed a different morphology from those stimulated by laminin indicating that specific ECM-receptor binding may activate different cytoskeletal components within the glioma cells [9]. It is further to such conceptual performance of mirror portrayal that the glioma cells further include the emergence of vascular structures as projected perivascular basement membranes, and as systems of mesenchymal structures pertinent to high grade gliomas. It is within the system projections for the realized infiltration of the brain parenchyma that the overall dimensions for growth of the parental tumor mass further incorporate systems of induced reproducibility of further enhancing infiltrative systems. AMPA receptors enhance perivascular glioma invasion via beta1 integrin-dependent adhesion to the ECM [10].

The integrins and the hyaluronan receptor CD44 are specific adhesion receptors involved in glioma-ECM adhesion; they also interact with the proteases secreted during glioma progression that allow tumor cells to diffusely infiltrate the CNS [11].

The incremental involvement of the central nervous system (CNS) as substitute for the primary tumor mesenchymal stroma is evidential realization of an increasing dimension for spread in terms of the growth of the parental tumor. The whole focus for adhesion molecules constitutes, as such, evidential components that allow for a permissive microenvironment that evolves as infiltrating glioma cells. New targets against glioma invasion include upstream mediators for cell adhesion, matrix degradation and cytoskeletal rearrangement [12]. It is significant to include the emergence of the distributive potential for spread as a conformational mirror image of such primary tumor within the system profile for further evolving dynamics. The performance of mirror imaging is projected as systems of portrayal and also as induction phenomena that signify the performance of attribute determination and predetermination of the inherent tumor biology systems. Glioblastomas appear to opt for the unfolded protein response to allow their continued uncontrolled growth by enhanced protein production and lipid biosynthesis [13].

PERFORMANCE REQUISITES

Performance requisites are biology of the primal malignant transformation process within the conceptual requirements of a process of reproducibility of such malignant transformation process in the infiltrating glioma cell bed of surgically resected tumors.

It is within systems of inherent hierarchical performance that the whole dimensional field of tumor growth and spread invokes the further conformational increments in tumor biology systems. The induction of epithelial mesenchymal transition (EMT) increases the invasiveness of various types of carcinoma but the role of transforming growth factor-beta (TGFbeta) remains to be elucidated in glioblastomas [14]. It is significant to view such realization as mirror-provocative systems of induction, as carried forward by adhesion molecule biology. Versican isoform 1 modulates proliferation and migration in high-grade gliomas; TGFbeta2 modulates glioma invasion and interacts with versican isoforms V0/V1 during malignant progression of glioma in vitro [15]. Possible connections between laminin-stimulated cell migration and the epidermal growth factor receptor expression may occur on glioma cells [16].

Significant carry-over phenomena of reproducible malignancy are further conformational crysallization of events that incorporates the overall confines of an infiltrating tumor edge. In such terms, the emergence of integrin confines of a given glioma is the emergence of significant inducing malignancy that portrays the biology of the parental tumor lesion. The contributing formulas, as projected by the infiltrating tumor edge, signify the emergence of attributes of conforming geometry as determined by the adjacent infiltrated brain parenchyma.

Conclusion

The significant object of reproducible malignant change in terms of the infiltrating tumor edge is beset by mesenchymal attributes of the adhesion molecules that empower dimensions of realization of mirror-image performance of such malignant change. It is further to such concepts that the emergence of projecting profiles of adhesion molecules induces the inhibitory attributes of adhesion molecules and also performs a concrete predetermination as confirmed by mirror-image profiles in their own right. The further conformations of malignancy are significant within spheroidal dimensions of geometric predetermination in their own right. The projection of such performance profiles includes the emergence of individuality of the tumor cell as portrayed by integrity of the whole parental tumor lesion. Hence, the mirror-image of primary tumors allows for a projection that is induced malignancy, as projected by systems of adhesion molecular biology subsets.

References

[1] Shimizu T, Kurozumi K, Ishida J, Ishikawa T, Date I "Adhesion molecules and the extracellular matrix as drug targets for glioma" *Brain Tumor Pathol* 2016;33(2):97-106.

[2] Venkatesh HSm Tan LT, Woo PJ, Lennon J, Nagaraja S, Gillespie SM et al. "Targeting neuronal activity-regulated neuroligin-3 dependency in high-grade glioma" *Nature* 2017;549(7673):533-537.

[3] Jiang Q, Xie Q, Hu C, Yang Z, Huang P, Shen H et al. "Glioma malignancy is linked to interdependent and inverse AMOG and L1 adhesion molecule expression" *BMC Cancer* 2019;19(1):911.

[4] Caldwell WT, de Tribolet N, Antel JP, Gauthier T, Kipper MC "Adhesion molecules and malignant gliomas: implications for tumorigenesis" *J Neurosurg* 1002;76(5):782-91.

[5] Liu N, Yang C, Bai W, Wang Z, Wang X, Johnson M et al. "CAM2 inhibits human glioma proliferation, migration and invasion" *Oncol Rep* 2019;41(4):2273-2280.

[6] Onishi M, Ishikawa T, Kurozumi K, Date I "Angiogenesis and invasion in glioma" *Brain Tumor Pathol* 2011;28(1):13-24.

[7] Goldbrunner RH, Bernstein JJ, Tonn JC "ECM-mediated glioma cell invasion" *Microsc Res Tech* 1998;43(3):250-7.

[8] Giese A, Laube B, Zapf S, Mangold U, Westphal M "Glioma cell adhesion and migration on human brain sections" *Anticancer Res;* 18(4A):2435-47.

[9] Mahesparan R, Tysnes BB, Edvardsen K, Haugeland HK, Cabrera IG, Lund-Johansen M et al. "Role of high molecular weight extracellular matrix proteins in glioma cell migration" *Neuropathol Appl Neurobiol* 1997;23(2):102-12.

[10] Piao Y, Lu L, de Groot J "AMPA receptors promote perivascular glioma invasion via beta1 integrin-dependent adhesion to the extracellular matrix" *Neuro Ocol* 2009;11(3):260-73.

[11] Bellail AC, Hunter SB, Brat D, Tan C, Van Meir EG "Microregional extracellular matrix heterogeneity in brain modulates glioma cell invasion" *Int J Biochem Cell Biol* 36(6):1046-69.

[12] Munson J, Bonner M, Fried L, Hofmekler J, Arisier J, Bellamkonda R "Identifying new small molecule anti-invasive compounds for glioma treatment" *Cell Cycle* 2013;12(14):2200-9.

[13] Graner MW "The unfolded protein response in glioblastomas: targetable or trouble?" *Future Sci OA* 2015;1(2):FSO45.

[14] Bryukhovetskiy I, Shevchenko V "Molecular mechanisms of the effect of TGF-beta1 on U87 human glioblastoma cells" *Oncol Lett* 2016;12(2):1581-1590.

[15] Oaken J, Moeckel S, Leukel P, Leidgens V, Baumann F, Bogdahn U et al. "Versican isoform V1 regulates proliferation and migration in high-grade gliomas" *J Neurooncol* 2014;120(1):73-83.

[16] Tysnes BB, Haugland HK, Berkvig R "Epidermal growth factor and laminin receptors contribute to migratory and invasive properties of gliomas" *Invasion Metastasis* 1007;17(5):270-80.

Chapter 5

FAILED TUMOR IMMUNO-ANTIGENICITY IS EXPRESSED SUPPRESSION OF AN AUTOIMMUNITY IN DEFINING IMMUNE PRIVILEGE STATUS OF THE LESION

ABSTRACT

System profiles of tumor antigenicity are real models of presented constitution within the cooperative participation of a suppressed autoimmune response to the neoplastic cells. It is significant to view the immune privileged status of the neoplastic lesion as substantial redefinition models as projected in terms of a blind immune response. The simplification modules of induction towards tumor cells, and the integral tumor lesion, allow for the emergence of lymphocytes that fail to recognize neoantigens as terms of provoked suppression of the autoimmune response.

Evasion of tumor cells from immunosurveillance is a complex group of strategies within the confined locus phenomenon of tumors that are simultaneous locally categorized and also spreading metastatic lesions. In this sense, the ongoing dynamics of tumor cell evasion utilize a huge repertoire of mechanisms that are persistently active during the processes of tumor cell growth and proliferation, and especially in the induction of both early and advanced stages of tumor metastatic spread.

Introduction

Substantial model representations of immune evasion appear, to some extent, centered on induced apoptosis of T lymphocytes; in other cases defects in major histocompatibility complex (MHC) antigenicity relate chiefly through a quasi-universal phenomenon of defective antigen presentation in terms of suppressed tumor antigenicity. Antibodies that block the immune checkpoint receptors PD1 and CTLA4 have revolutionised the treatment of melanoma and many other cancers; this therapeutic blockade of inhibitory receptors breaks self-tolerance and highlights a crucial role in the physiologic modulation of the immune response [1]. The overall dimensions of antigen presentation are involved participation of tumor cell immunogenicity as terms of reference within system dynamics of multi -agent operability.

Regulatory T cells (Treg) are implicated in tumor development and progression by inhibiting antitumor immunity; a high infiltration by Treg cells is associated with poor survival in various types of cancer [2].

Consequential participation is therefore required in the face of tumor neoantigenicity as far evolved within terms of ongoing antigen presentation. It is within the scope involvement of immune privilege dynamics that the primary and metastatic lesions prove resistant to an immune response by host lymphocytes and by natural killer cells.

The progression of tumor cell biologic variability is consistent with an evolutionary course directly dependent on such immune privileged status of the individual tumor cells and also of the whole tumor lesion. It seems mandatory to stop immunosuppressive or immunomodulating agents during radiotherapy [3].

Interactivity

In terms of ongoing interactivities of lymphocytes towards immune attack on tumor and tumor cells, the evolutionary nature of ongoing involvement of a defective antigen presentation participates as genetic mutability and as substantial involvement of antigen transport and processing within different classes of cell type.

INTERPLAY DYNAMICS

Participating interplay includes the various different dimensions of interactivity between tumor cells and homing lymphocytes. The distinctive profiles of such interactivity are lack of recognition of the tumor specific antigens as brought forward by the dendritic cell network. Antigen presentation is hence a centrally dominant phenomenon in its own right that in addition is independently operative and distinct from tumor cell dynamics. It is in terms of a realized contrast confrontation that there evolves system definition as network co-operability and modulation. The ongoing characterization of lymphocytes consists of the privileged status of expression of MHC/Peptide complexes at the surface of the cell.

In this sense, the evolutionary dimensions of cooperative modulations of the immune response are distinct in terms of tumor antigenicity and immunogenicity.

It is further to such defining terms, that ongoing tumor antigenicities are relatively operative factors in the defined modulation of the immune system, as specifically characterized by an active immune-privileged status. Extracellular vesicles from both non-immune and immune cells are important in immune regulation [4].

VARIABILITY OF ANTIGENICITY

Variability of antigenicity as offered by the tumor cells is cardinal participant in the modulated immune response to such tumor cells. Immunosuppressed patients are at increased risk of developing cutaneous cancer [5]. The ongoing definitions of the immune-privileged status of tumors are a representation of imaged ignorance in terms that go beyond lymphocyte interactivity. Neutrophils are key drivers of cancer progression and affect proliferation, aggressiveness and dissemination of tumors as well as immune suppression [6]. It is as systems of network operability that there evolves a state of tolerance and of anergy within the tumor cell operabilities as primarily spreading lesions. The roles of metastatic lesions in such interplay are illustrative within the network cooperation of antigen-presenting cells in such immune ignorance.

The system profile models are constitutive within the sphere of failed recognition status of the immune response, in the face of specific neoantigenicity of the tumor cells.

In terms of such a conceptual definition of the dimensions of tumor induced immune privilege, the ongoing frontiers of the constitutive tumor lesion are active modulators of the central immunogenicity governing the immune response as integral networks. Myasthenia Gravis can manifest as a paraneoplastic disorder in the context of a thymoma [7].

Lymphocyte Non-Reactivity

The provocative systems of lymphocyte activation by tumor cell neoantigenicity are therefore a core phenomenon that fails within the encompassed profile participation of tissue injury recognition. In terms of different dimensional definition of the immune response, the emergence of such immune response is ineffective as systems of basic reactivity. The composite reformulation of such immune response is further projected within the pathway promotional definition as terms of model decoy processes of suppressed immunogenicity.

The interplay systems for further progression of the tumor pathobiology are hence central to the initial carcinogenesis events as portrayed by the systems of network operability and co-operability.

It is in the terms of such network participation, that the suppressed autoimmunity, as presented by the tumor lesion, arises as factors of modulated further involvement of the failed immune response. It is, furthermore, clearly within dimensional versatility of antigen presentation that the defining terms of the immune privileged status emerges.

The significance of a suppressed autoimmunity is relative phenomenon as projected by the variability profiles of different tumor antigens presented to professional antigen-presenting cells such as dendritic cells. Helminth parasite infection may potentially reduce tumor immunosurveillance and also reduce vaccine response [8].

Systems of Processing

Participating systems of processing of antigens are dependent on the intracellular transport systems as conveying participants that are directed towards the delivery of protein peptides to the lumen of the endoplasmic reticulum. The further promotional terms of participation of the MHC molecular assembly allow for the ignorant immune response as projected by defective tumor antigen presentation. The whole process is hence the contrasting suppressive events with regard to the universal autoimmune status of cells and tissue organs. Immune checkpoint inhibitors and small-molecule targeted drugs have significantly improved patient prognosis in patients with metastatic cutaneous melanoma [9].

It is simple suppressive modulation of an otherwise emerging autoimmunity that a formulated definition of suppression of the immune system is realized. The immune system ensures optimum T-effector immune responses against invading microbes and tumor antigens while preventing inappropriate autoimmune responses with the help of T-regulatory cells [10].

Immune Priviliged Status

Hence, in restricted terms of operability, the immune-privileged status of the tumor cells and of the integral tumor lesion is a permissive series of roles of suppression as lymphocytes, such as cytotoxic lymphocytes, fail to actively kill the neoplastic cells and tissues. In a sense, the angiogenesis and reactive tumor stromal elements are expressive phenomena as projected by an early event in acquisition of spreading metastatic potential by the neoplasm.

CONCLUSION

Ongoing involvement as portrayed by an immune-privileged status of tumor cells is resultant facet within a suppressed autoimmunity as otherwise provoked by tumor cell neoantigenicity. Immune checkpoint signaling dampens T cell activation to prevent autoimmunity [11]. In such terms, ongoing profiles of modeled presentation of antigen by neoplastic cells are defining terms of a failed autoimmune response. Significant characterization of such series of events is projected in terms of a realization of the immune response itself to the tumor cell neoantigenicity, as portrayed in patient host reactivity to foreign antigens in general.

Recent observations in cancer clinical trials using blocking antibodies against PD-1 or/and CTLA4 have shown a high incidence of autoimmune-related side-effects and illustrate the important role of these pathways in human immune homeostasis [12].

REFERENCES

[1] Paluch C, Santos AM, Anzilotti C, Cornall RJ, Davis SJ "Immune checkpoints as therapeutic targets in autoimmunity" *Front Immunol* 2018;9:2306.

[2] Ohue Y, Nishikawa H "Regulatory T (Treg) cells in cancer: can Treg cells be a new therapeutic target?" *Cancer Sci* 2019;110(7):2080-2089.

[3] Basacki C, Vallard A, Jmour O, Ben Mrad M, Lahmamssi C, Bousarsar A et al. "Radiotherapy and immune suppression: a short review" *Bull Cancer* 2020;107(1):84-101.

[4] Robbins PD, Morelli AE "Regulation of immune responses by extracellular vesicles" *Nat Rev Immunol* 2014/14(3):195-208.

[5] Collins L, Quinn A, Stasko T "Skin cancer and immunosuppression" *Dermal Clin* 2019;37(1):83-94.

[6] Lecot P, Sarabi M, Pereira Abrantes M, Mussard J, Koenderman L, Caux C et al. "Neutrophil Heterogeneity in cancer: from biology to therapies" *Front Immunol* 2019;10:2155.

[7] Mullges W, Stoll G "Myasthenia gravis" *Nervenarzt* 2019;90(10):1055-1066.

[8] Maizels RM, McSorley HJ "Regulation of the host immune system by helminth parasites" *J Allergy Clin Immunol* 2016;138(3):666-675.

[9] Pasquali S, Hadjinicolaou AV, Chiarion Sileni V, Rossi CR, Mocellin S "Systemic treatments for metastatic cutaneous melanoma" *Cochrane Database Syst Rev* 2018;2(2):CD011123.

[10] Kumar P, Bhattacharya P, Prabhakar BS "A comprehensive review on the role of co-signaling receptors and Treg homeostasis in autoimmunity and tutor immunity" *J Autoimmun* 2018;95:77-99.

[11] Pico de Coana Y, Chowdhury A, Kiessling R "Checkpoint blockade for cancer therapy: revitalising a suppressed immune system" *Trends Mol Med* 2015;21(8):482-91.

[12] Murakami N, Riella LV "Co-inhibitory pathways and their importance in immune regulation" *Transplantation* 2014;98(1):3-14.

Chapter 6

COMPLEX EFFECTIVENESS OF GENERAL IMMUNITY IN MODULATING THE SPECIFIC IMMUNE RESPONSE IN GLIOMAS

ABSTRACT

Construed determinants within immune reactivity frameworks allow a permissive microenvironment of high grade gliomas to participate within systems of modulated response in terms of targeting events. The significance for reproduction of glioma attributes is system specification as determined by dynamics of a generalized systemic response of such modulated immunity. The participation of injury to the individual glioma cell is further projected within frameworks of such reappraisal as evidenced by emergence of the glioma lesion per se, and as further targeting of an immune response specified by dynamics of proliferation and spread of high grade glioma cells intracranially.

INTRODUCTION

The conceptual framework for the development of immune response to intracranial gliomas constitutes a realization that potential attack involvement is a prerogative of immune reactivity in general terms. The ultimate success of immunotherapy in the central nervous system (CNS) depends on improved imaging technologies and analysis of the tumor microenvironment [1]. Evidence suggests that vaccine strategies, such as the dendritic cell, heat shock protein or EGFRvIII vaccines may provide promise for promoting immunogenicity [2]. It is also reasonable to consider the derivative dimensions of antigen presentation as an attribute that determines a whole spectrum of reactivities within the further development of autoimmunity on the one hand and the traditional concepts of immune privilege of the central nervous system. Emerging themes indicate the importance of mitigating the immunosuppressive tumor microenvironment and the potential for innate immune cell activation to enhance cytotoxic anti-tumor activity [3]. It is indeed relevant to consider derivative dimensions of immune reactivity as a plural phenomenon as dictated by heterogeneity of high grade gliomas in general. Major types of immunotherapy include vaccines, cell-based therapies, and immune checkpoint modulators for glioblastoma [4].

Antigen Presentation

The distributive biology of antigen presentation within the CNS confirms the further potentiality for development of concepts of biology of the immune response, as borne out by systems of enhanced reproducibility of specific dimensions in the immune response as evidenced by glioma biology. Tumors require a re-analysis of currently accepted treatment strategies as well as newly designed approaches [5].

The conclusive dimensions of operability are clearly the immune suppressive attributes of the CNS as partial immune privilege of the CNS. Multiple immunosuppressive mechanisms and micro-invasion result in a complex interplay glioblastoma shares with the immune system [6]. In such terms, the strict experimental confirmation of immune responsiveness to glioma cell proliferation and spread is further defined by systems of response especially of T helper cells on the one hand and of cytotoxic T cells on the other.

Immune System Specificity

Autologous stimulated lymphocytes, cytokines and dendritic cells, immune checkpoint inhibitors, virotherapy and tumor or peptide based vaccines are promising therapies [7].

Genetics and epigenetics of glioblastoma have revealed aberrations in cellular signaling pathways, the tumor microenvironment and pathologic angiogenesis [8].

The potential specificity of the immune response to high grade gliomas is thus a re-evaluation of indices for Major Histocompatibility Complex performance as determined specifically by antigen-presenting cells including microglia and endothelial cells in particular. The future of therapy for glioblastoma will probably involve a combinatorial personalised approach utilizing conventional treatments, active immunotherapeutics, and agents targeting immunosuppressive check points [9].

The distributive dynamics of response as dictated by lymphocytes, macrophages and antigen-presenting cells allow for transformation of an essential permissive micro-environment within systems of ongoing response to foreign antigens. The further cooperative functionality of the intracranial immune response bespeaks for the unfolding redistribution of lymphocytes found in regions of perivascular spaces, cerebrospinal fluid, and also ependyma and choroid plexus. In such dimensions, reproducibility and recurrence of a robust immune response clearly indicate enhancement potentiality as borne out by systems of reproducibility of immunity as further portrayed by reactivated memory immune cell components.

Potential Dynamics

Inclusive dimensions for potential dynamics are substantive component derivation is simple reconstitution of an immune response that further redefines the nature of the intracranial immune response.

Checkpoint blockade induces anti-tumor activity by preventing negative regulation of T-cell activation; checkpoint block is probably most effective in combination with a dendritic vaccine or adoptively transferred tumor-specific T cells generated ex vivo [10].

The conclusive recovery of such immune response is phylogenetically a derivative natural attribute of the immune system both systemically and intracranially. In such terms, the development of injury and degeneration of actively proliferating and spread of high grade glioma cells is system determined agonistic action within redefined homeostasis and dyshomeostasis of the immune reactivity.

Series of Reactivities

It is further to such considerations that a full repertoire of reactivities on the part of the immune system redefines the nature of immunity in general terms. It is significant to consider the further confirmatory evidence as projected by systems of modulation of biologic attributes of the cytotoxic CD8+ lymphocyte subsets.

Immunotherapeutic classes under investigation include vaccination strategies, adoptive T cell immunotherapy, immune checkpoint blockade, monoclonal antibodies and cytokine therapies [11].

Receptivity expression on lymphocytes on the one hand and on glioma cells attests for the potential reproduction of immune responses within frameworks of attributes within systems of ongoing transformation. Micro RNAs have been implicated in glioma initiation and progression and miR-1254 inhibits progression in vivo and vitro of glioma by targeting Colony Stimulating Factor-1 [12].

The persistence of redistribution of lymphocytes within the CNS further attests to an evolutionary series of courses that biologically implicate the immune response. The considerable dimensions for change are dictated strictly by both general immune responsiveness and of also specific immune reactivity to antigens on the surface of glioma cells and of internal determinants within the tumor cells. Optimal implementation in immunotherapy of glioblastoma may depend on familiarity with tumor specific antigens presented as HLA peptides by the glioblastoma cells [13].

By such conceptual determination of the reactive immune response, the overall generalized immunity is specific expression in terms of reactive attack to the dynamics of tumor cell proliferation and spread intracranially.

IMMUNE RESPONSE INCREMENTS

Powerful increments in the immune response implicate complement production and action within the milieu of adjuvant co-stimulation of the antigenicity of the individual glioma cell. In such terms, the distributive dynamics of the endothelial cells further attest to potentially strong reactivities of prioritization of the general immune response as dictated in terms beyond simple frameworks of the specific immune reactivities. Escape from immunosurveillance is increasingly recognised as a landmark event in cancer biology; glioblastoma has emerged as a model of resistance to immunotherapy [14]. It is beyond such terms that derivational predominance of the general immunity systems of reappraisal implicates a second wave of specific immunity states that determines survival and death of the individual glioma cell in particular.

Significant reappraisal for transformed dynamics of immune response indicate a system modulation as potential dimension for the induction of specific targeting as borne out by modulation on the part by a general immunity response to such antigens as epidermal growth factor variant III.

It is to be further realized that the overall conformational antigenicity of the high grade glioma cells is system modulation of the general immune responsiveness in the overall dynamics of reproducibility of specific attack on the individual glioma cell. Immunotherapy via adoptive cell transfer especially offers T cells engineered to express chimeric antigen receptors; primary immunologic challenges in glioblastoma implicate antigenic heterogeneity, immune suppression and T-cell exhaustion [15].

Biology of Immunity

Biology of immune responsiveness is a question of attribute specification within the ongoing immune reactivity patterns that modulate and further shape antigenicity as presented by glioma cells to generalized immune system function and dysfunction. In such terms, the systemic dysfunctions of the immune response preselects targeted rejection of the glioma cells as determined in particular by both microglia and dendritic cells found within the neural parenchyma. It is significant to reconsider complement and co-stimulatory molecules as derived redistribution of a series of pathways for further modulation of the immune responsiveness. Research addressing synergism between treatment options is gaining attention [16].

Antigen presentation is a biologic framework for both generalized and specific immune targeting of the individual glioma cell that is actively undergoing both proliferation and spread intracranially. Neoadjuvant anti-programmed cell death protein 1 immunotherapy enhances survival benefit with intratumoral and systemic immune responses in recurrent glioblastoma [17]. The redistributive dimensions of glioma biology is significant reappraisal for further conformation restructuring of the immune response itself. It is within such framework that the characterization of glioma antigenicity conforms to the emergence of the glioma cell as experienced by proliferation and spread of such individual glioma cell.

Conclusion

Complex formulation of incremental nature is a strict requisite to the ongoing potential targeting of the glioma cells as derived immune responsiveness to specific determinants created by active proliferation and spread of the individual glioma cell.

Such redistribution of antigenicity is determinant functionality as projected by a general or systemic immune responsiveness that derives and further develops a secondary specificity of the immune response that is carried forward by systems of modulation of the cytotoxic CD8+ lymphocyte subset. Performance indices of such reappraisal are dysfunctional and specific cooperative target creation within the pathway evolution to the immunity phenomena of the glioma cells that undergo proliferation and spread intracranially.

REFERENCES

[1] Sampson JH, Maus MV, June CH "Immunotherapy for brain tumors" *J Clin Oncol* 2017;35(21):2450-2456.

[2] Schernberg A, Marabelle A, Massard C, Armand JP, Dumont S, Deutsch E et al. "What's next in glioblastoma treatment: timor-targeted or immune-targeted therapies?" *Bull Cancer* 2016;103(5):484-98.

[3] Lieberman NAP, Moyes KW, Crane CA "Developing immunotherapeutic strategies to target brain tumors" *Expert Rev Anticancer There* 2016;16(7):775-88.

[4] Reardon DA, Wen PY, Wucherpfennig KW, Sampson JH "Immunomodulation for glioblastoma" *Curr Opin Neurol* 2017;30(3):361-369.

[5] Wainwright DA, Nigam P, Thaci B, Dey M, Lesniak M "Recent developments on immunotherapy for brain cancer" *Expert Opin Emerg Drugs* 2012;17(2):181-202.

[6] Cohen-Inbar O, Zaaroor M "Immunological aspects of malignant gliomas" *Can J Neural Sci* 2016;43(4):494-502.

[7] Weathers SP, Gilbert MR "Current challenges in designing GBM trials for immunotherapy" *J Neurooncol* 2016;123(3):331-7.

[8] Polka J Jr, Polka J, Holubec L, Kubikova T, Priban V, Hes O et al. "Advances in experimental targeted therapy and immunotherapy for

patients with glioblastoma multiforme" *Anticancer Res* 2017;37(1):21-33.

[9] Huang B, Zhang H, Gu L, Ye B, Zhihong J, Stary C et al. "Advances in immunotherapy for glioblastoma multiforme" *J Immunol Res* 2017;2017:3697613.

[10] Desai R, Suryadevara CM, Batich KA, Farber SH, Sanchez-Perez L, Sampson JH "Emerging immunotherapies for glioblastoma" *Expert Opin Emerg Drugs* 2016;21(2):133-45.

[11] Harrison Farber S, Elsamadicy AA, Atik AF, Suryadevara CM, Chongsathidkiet P, Facci PE et al. "The safety of available immunotherapy for the treatment of glioblastoma" *Expert Opin Drug Saf* 2017;16(3):277-287.

[12] Li X, Kong S, Cao Y "miR-1254 inhibits progression of glioma in vivo and in vitro by targeting CSF-1" *J Cell Mol Med* 2020;24(5):3128-3138.

[13] Shraibman B, Barnea E, Kadosh DM, Haimovich Y, Slobodan G, Rosner I et al. "Identification of tumor antigens among the HLA peptidomes of glioblastoma tutors and plasma" *Mol Cell Proteomics* 2019;18(6):1255-1268.

[14] Jackson CM, Choi J, Lim M "Mechanisms of immunotherapy resistance: lessons from glioblastoma" *Nat Immmul* 2019;20(9):1100-1109.

[15] Choi BD, Maus MV, June CH, Sampson JH "Immunotherapy for glioblastoma: adoptive T-cell strategies" *Clin Cancer Res* 2019;25(7):2042-2048.

[16] Miyauchi JT, Tsirka SE "Advances in immunotherapeutic research for glioma therapy" *J Neural* 2018;265(4):741-756.

[17] Cloughesy TF, Mochizuki A, Orpilla JR, Hugo W, Lee AH, Davidson TB et al. "Neoadjuvant anti-PD-1 immunotherapy promotes a survival benefit with intratumoral and systemic immune responses in recurrent glioblastoma" *Nat Med* 2019;25(3):477-586.

Chapter 7

SYSTEMS OF MALIGNANT TRANSFORMATION AS INTEGRAL IMMUNE NONRESPONSE IN GLIOMAGENESIS

ABSTRACT

Dynamics of establishment of gliomagenesis both outline and further extend the provoked induction of injury to local groups of glial cells within the encompassed malignant transformation events. Tonic and phasic participants as realized by systems of provoked induction support an infiltrativeness that redefines the nature of the actively infiltrated, surrounding, pseudo-normal brain tissues in general. In such terms, provoked malignant transformation is system pathway definition within the realization of a phasic/tonic alteration of adoptive systems of induced further non-response of the immune system. As supportive increments for further change this is projected as the malignant transformation phenomenon.

INTRODUCTION

Insofar that it is possible to consider the directional phase construction of malignant gliomas within encompassed development of the malignant transformation process, it is also true to consider evolutionary dynamics as central to such malignant transformation. Functional enrichment analysis and protein-protein interaction networks have shown differential expression of genes mainly implicated in immune response, cell adhesion and extracellular matrix [1]. It is to be realized that the outcome mechanisms of the malignant transformation constitutes a series of induced parameters that outstrip normal adjustments of growth and proliferative systems as further dynamics of tumor outcome at initial stages of inception of the lesion. In such terms, the development of injury to glial cells is an inherent susceptibility of glial cells in general, with the added improviso that malignant change of glial cells is a cardinal and central issue that reflects the process of carcinogenesis in general as it applies to human patients.

Present evidence indicates that tumor infiltration by lymphocytes can be generated by dendritic cell immunotherapy and this may influence clinical outcome [2]. Several glioma-derived factors trigger migration, accumulation and re-programming of immune-competent cells [3].

Injury to Glial Cells

The development of injury in genesis is a feature of gliomagenesis within the further conformational dynamics of cell replacement. CD155 plays an important role in anti-glial immune responses and is a promising immunotherapy target [4]. In such conceptual framework, the further evolution of such injury is central to a lesion that is non-adaptively concerned with the secretion of immunosuppressive molecules such as transforming growth factor beta (TGF-beta). With such evolution, the adoption of glial cell injury is paramount consideration in the re-directional proliferation and spread of malignant cells that arise and further progress as dynamics of such proliferation and spread within the central nervous system. Future clinical trials need to consider the diversity constituted by high-grade glioma especially in the paediatric population [5]. It is also indicated that the whole series of transforming immune reactivities against the malignant glioma cells is inherent dynamics of the initial injury event as terms of phasic reconstitution of such injured glial cells.

On the evidence afforded by a variety of potential biomarkers of response to immune checkpoints, only minor subsets of glioma patients are likely to benefit from mono-therapy immune checkpoint inhibition [6].

PERFORMANCE OF TUMORS

Performance residual is a conceptual framework that affords gliomas in general but especially lesions such as glioblastoma as referential systems of a gliomagenesis fully dependent on intense angiogenesis as especially portrayed by glioblastoma. It is further to such considerations that gliomas both portray and further extend the scope of the malignant transformation series of events that primarily infiltrate and only secondarily proliferate. It is towards the inception of such infiltration that the development of further glial cell injury conformationally modifies the immune response as well illustrated by TGF-beta actions.

Tumor infiltrating lymphocytes and programmed death ligand 1 are targets of immune checkpoint inhibitors; IDH -wt gliomas display a more prominent TIL infiltration and higher PD-L1 expression than IDH-mut cases [7].

The inhibition of activation of T- cells as evidenced by the TGF-beta action is a phase dynamics within the system pathway as portrayed by systems of immune non-responsiveness.

The emergence of such malignant transformation hence arises as dynamics of immune nonresponse in the first instance, and as dynamics further projected within spheres of involvement of the initial injury phase of in situ glial cells in general. The profiling of Neurofibromatosis 1-glioma defines a distinct landscape that recapitulates a subset of sporadic tumors [8]. It is such conceptual involvement of the outcome evolutionary phases of involvement that the development of inducible injury further invokes the progression of the malignant glioma as strictly defined in terms of exchange and reconstitutive processes as delivered by the surrounding brain tissues that undergo processes of phasic infiltration by tumor cells. The proportions of several immune cells are significantly related to patient age and sex; also the level of M0 macrophages is significant in regard to interactions with other immune cells, including monocytes and gamma delta T cells [9].

INDUCTION OF MALADAPTATION

Induced maladaptive phenomena are the projected generic substantial responsiveness as further provoked by the malignant transformational process. In such terms, the outcome of initial injury is phasic dynamics as provoked by the replacement of the normal cellular structure of the CNS as evidenced by infiltrative behavior of the malignant glioma.

It is further considered realization that the outcome initial determination for further transformation is central paramount consideration of the subsequent phases of infiltration of normal brain tissues. Further provoked increments in the growth of a malignant glioma are supportive transformation of immunosuppressive molecules such as TGF-beta as particularly secreted by the neoplastic glioma cells themselves.

In the glioma microenvironment, Toll-like receptor 2 activation of microglia induces down regulation of microglial MHC class II expression and this limits T-cell-dependent antitumor immunity [10].

Juxta-positional arrangements of infiltrating glioma cells are modifications as further portrayed by phasic adjustments in terms also of tonic realizations of the initial injury. This is further projected as phasic component pathways in glioma genesis. It is such susceptibility dynamics that constitute the further adaptive adoption of an injurious glioma cell within systems of induction for further evolutionary course. The performance of the outcome development of gliomagenesis are intrinsic attributes for further transformations in image evolution of the whole process of infiltrative involvement of the brain.

Proportional Correlates

Proportional correlates of the infiltration of glioma cells are hence a failure of the immune responses as further modified by manipulative dimensions of intense proliferation of the neoplastic cells. Pilot data has shown that adding intratumor injection of dendritic cells extends survival of patients with glioblastoma treated by subcutaneous delivery of dendritic cells [11]. In such conceptual frameworks of phasic and tonic constructs of nonresponse of the immune system, the outcome dynamics of malignant transformation both realize and further potentiate the dynamics of proliferation of the tumor cells within systems for further infiltration of emerging modifications of the pseudo-normal brain tissues. In such terms, the outcome dynamics are maladjustments within systems of alternating response and nonresponse of the immune system, in part or as a whole phase of incremental intensity. Studies have shown the safety and antitumor effects of autologous tumor lysate-pulsed dendritic cell therapy for patients with malignant glioma [12].

Infiltrated Brain Tissues

The defining terms as projected by infiltrated brain tissue are modified phase constructs of a system of immune non-development within systems of genetic injury to glial cells and glioma cells.

In such terms, the further conformational adoption of such genetic injury is itself a reflection of the system pathway confirmation of the system targeting that may act both phasically and tonically to the realization of progression of the malignant gliomagenesis. Targeting pathways are analytic tools within the malignant transformation events that progress within the confined limits of local processing as evidenced by biology of adhesion molecules in surrounding brain tissues.

Such considerations are indicative of a permissiveness that promotes the dissemination of tumor cells in terms of strict localization events within transforming tissues. It is further to such considerations that the transforming events themselves strictly define the nature of the initial injury to glial cells and the concurrent nonresponse of the immune system to the transforming malignant events. Vaccination of patients with high-grade glioma with peptide-pulsed dendritic cells enhances systemic cytotoxicity and intracranial T-cell infiltration [13].

The future likely resides in combinatorial approaches, with administration of surgery and radiochemotherapy and immunotherapy once schedules for treatment are established [14]. Dendritic cell vaccines, adoptive cell transfer, and oncolytic viruses may potentially play a role in the treatment of patients with malignant glioma [15].

Thanks to recent advancements in cell engineering technologies, infusion of ex vivo prepared immune cells have emerged as promising strategies of cancer immunotherapy [16].

Conclusion

Dynamics of phase replacement of the surrounding brain tissue indicate a real series of substitutions of the malignant transformation phase as further projected in terms of infiltrativeness. In such defined scope, the performance emergence of injury is substantial redefinition of the immune nonresponsiveness that is realized as projected amplifying genetic injury in the transforming glioma cells. It is further to such considerations that the paramount proliferative rates of tumor cells come to dominate a phasic and tonic series of infiltrativeness that is unique to the transformation event per se and as established earmark of the malignancy that provokes further immune suppression.

References

[1] Jia D, Li S, Li D, Xue H, Yang D, Liu Y "Mining TCGA database for genes of prognostic value in glioblastoma microenvironment" *Aging* (Albany NY) 2018;10(4):592-605.

[2] Sokratous G, Polyzoidis S, Ashkan K "Immune infiltration of tumor microenvironment following immunotherapy for glioblastoma multiforme" *Hum Vaccin Immunother* 2017;13(11):2575-2582.

[3] Gieryng A, Pszczolkowska D, Walentynowicz KA, Rajan WD, Kaminska B "Immune microenvironment of gliomas" *Lab Invest* 2017;97(5):498-518.

[4] Liu F, Huang J, Xiong Y, Li S, Liu Z "Large-scale analysis reveals the specific clinical and immune features of CD155 in glioma" *Aging* (Albany NY) 2019;11(15):5463-5482.

[5] Mackay A, Burford A, Molinari V, Jones DTW, Izquierdo E, Brouwer-Visser J et al. "Molecular, pathological, radiological, and immune profiling of non-brainstem paediatric high-grade glioma from the HERBY phase II randomised trial" *Cancer Cell* 2018;33(5):829-842.

[6] Hodges TR, Ott M, Xiu J, Gatalica Z, Swensen J, Zhou S et al. "Mutational burden, immune checkpoint expression and mismatch repair in glioma: implications for immune checkpoint immunotherapy" *Neuro Oncol* 2017;19(8):1047-1057.

[7] Berghoff AS, Kiesel B, Lidhalm G, Wilhelm D, Rajky O, Kurscheid S et al. "Correlation of immune phenotype with IDH mutation in diffuse glioma" *Neuro Oncol* 2017;19(11):1460-1468.

[8] D'Angelo F, Ceccarelli M, Tala, Garofano L, Zhang J , Frattini V et al. "The molecular landscape of glioma in patients with Neurofibromatosis 1" *Nat Med* 2019;25(1):176-187.

[9] Zhong QY, Fan EX, Feng GY, Chen QY, Gou XX, Yue GJ et al. "A gene expression-based study on immune cell subtypes and glioma prognosis" *BMC Cancer* 2019;19(1):1116.

[10] Qian J, Luo F, Yang J, Liu J, Liu R, Wang L et al. "TLR2 promotes glioma immune evasion by down regulating MHC Class II molecules in microglia" *Cancer Immunol Res* 2018;6(10):1220-1233.

[11] Pellegatta S, Poliani PL, Stucchi E, Corno D, Colombo CA, Orzan F et al. "Intra-tumoral dendritic cells increase efficacy of peripheral vaccination by modulation of glioma microenvironment" *Neuro Oncol* 2010;12(4):377-88. 81.

[12] Yamanaka R, Abe T, Yakima N, Tsuchiya N, Homma J, Kobayashi T et al. "Vaccination of recurrent glioma patients with tutor lysate-pulsed dendritic cells elicits immune responses: results of a clinical phase I/II trial" *Br J Cancer* 2003;89(7):1172-9.

[13] Yu JS, Wheeler CJ, Zeltzer PM, Ying H, Finger DN, Lee PK et al. "Vaccination of malignant glioma patients with peptide-pulsed dendritic cells elicits systemic cytotoxicity and intracranial T-cell infiltration" *Cancer Res* 2001;61(3):842-7.

[14] De Carli E, Delion M, Rousseau A "Immunotherapy in brain tumours" *Ann Pathol* 2017;37(1):117-126.

[15] Maxwell R, Luksik AS, Garzon-Muvdi T, Lim M "The potential of cellular- and viral-based immunotherapies for malignant glioma—dendritic cell vaccines, adoptive cell transfer, and oncolytic viruses" *Curr Neural Neurosci Rep* 2017;17(6):50.

[16] Lin Y, Okada H "Cellular immunotherapy for malignant gliomas" *Expert Opin Biol There* 2016;16(10):1265-75.

Chapter 8

IMMUNODOMINANCE AS COMPLEX PATTERNED INTERPLAY OF ANTIGEN QUANTITATION PHENOMENA IN PRESSURE IMMUNITY

ABSTRACT

The basis of biology of immunodominance of antigens is defining term in the evolution of a specific antigenicity as carried forward by complex dimensions of an immune response to tumor epitopes. In such terms, immune pressure dynamics contextualize the evolving process of epitope redistribution as anergic states of nonreactivity or as terms of reference in defining such immunodominance of given antigenicity of individual tumor cells. It is further to such considerations that quantitative antigen presentation both correlates with evolution of antigen binding to the major histocompatiblity complex (MHC) structured molecules and with system profiles of redistribution inherent to antigen presentation on the surface membrane of both antigen presenting cells and also tumor cells.

Introduction

The immunodominance of given specific antigens is linked to the development of potentially robust immune response to tumors in general or to the emergence of profiles of reactivity of T cells in general. Neoadjuvant PD-1 immune checkpoint blockade reverses functional immunodominance amongst tumor antigen-specific T cells [1]. The complexities of immune response to neoplasms if further increased by antigen presentation phenomena inherently activate CD4+ and CD8+ T lymphocytes. Immunisation with in vitro selected cancer variants that lack the immunodominant antigen can disrupt the immunodominance and avoid escape of cancers from host immunity [2]. In such terms, the evolving redistribution of antigen epitopes is a potential series of mechanisms that dominants in various ways in regard to particular quantitative degrees of expression levels of specific antigen epitopes. Somatic mutations can induce cancer-specific neoepitopes there recognised by autologous T cells as foreign and constitute ideal cancer vaccine targets [3]. Hence, it may be relevant to consider the variability of heterogeneity of epitope antigenicity as provided not only by antigens among various different types of tumor but also heterogeneity of such antigen expression within the same neoplastic lesion.

Demarcation Profiles of Antigenicity

In conceptual terms, demarcation profiles between tumors or tumor types are system parameters with the biologic significance of the immune response to mitotically active infiltrating lesions. A significant fraction of non-synonymous cancer mutations is immunogenic and that most of the immunogenic mutanome is recognised by CD4+ T cells; mutational MHC class II epitopes drive therapeutic immune response to cancer [4]. In such terms, the explicit dimensions of increments in the immune response might arise within systems of immunodominance of given expressed epitopes. It is not known whether the human immune system often mounts a T cell response against motions expressed by epithelial cancers [5]. In the sense of evolutionary pressure phenomena the redistribution of antigenic profiles may allow for heterogeneous differentiation of various multiple clones of malignant tumor cells.

IMMUNODOMINANCE

Immunodominance is hence a redistribution of epitopes within actively growing neoplasms within the system biology attempts of immunosurveillance attempts in creating reactivity to given tumor cell clones within a given neoplasm and neoplasm type. Immunohistochemistry often appears to highlight the variability of epitope expression as projected by antigenicity profiles of a tumor. In a restrictive sense, the evolutionary emergence of particular epitope expression is beyond homeostatic control and is thus a biologically inherent attribute of reactivity as dimensionalized by T cell subtypes.

ANTIGENICITY

Poor degrees of antigenicity or non-expression of antigens are simple parametric emergence phenomena in the inherent activation mechanics of T lymphocytes. Immunodominance constitutes the breadth of antitumor T CD8 responses and is as such considered an impediment to effective vaccination against cancer [6]. The simple juxtaposition of given antigen moieties is enhanced redistribution of epitope specificity as dictated by systems of predominantly quantitative degrees of expressivity and of binding affinity of the given epitope. Mucin-associated sialyl-Tn antigens bind to receptors on dendritic cells, macrophages and natural killer cells that result in overall immunosuppression by receptor masking or inhibit of cytolytic ability [7].

Major histocompatibility complex binding is a system profile determinant within the biologic expressivity inherent to epitope presentation to T lymphocytes. Robust antitumor immune responses are induced in paediatric acute lymphoblastic leukaemia despite their low mutation burden and stress the importance of immunodominance in modulating cellular immune responses [8].

Expressivity of Antigen

Prominence of immunodominance is further contextual expressivity within the identity profile of the cell type origin of a specific tumor lesion and tumor histologic type. The evolving dimensions of tumor cell growth are determinants in terms of antigen loss phenomena on a clonal basis and on an individual tumor cell.

Potency of the specificity of antigen expression is secondary consideration of the activation phenomena of lymphocytes as projected within system biology of the molecular identity profiles as given expression of the immune response. Development of strategies that aim to enhance the total Tumor-associated antigens-specific CD8+ T cell response may be obtained by therapeutic boosting and/or specificity diversification [9]. The nature of molecular expression and of immune response bespeak of a whole series of complex interplay within the variability of anergic phenomena of various multiple complexes of antigenicity.

Treatment with interferon gamma, which up regulates the transcription of MHC class I is involved in antigen presentation and most of tutor lines are able to respond normally [10].

Antigen Identity

Identity of particular antigens in antigenicity studies allows for a possible reappraisal of system reactivities within the given dimensions of expressed antigen expression by tumor cell heterogeneity phenomena. To date, the alterations in the expression of MHC molecules play a critical role in tutor development due to defective antigen presentation to T-lymphocytes and regulation of natural killer cell function [11]. The redistribution of presented antigen epitopes is further complex consideration as terms of quantitative degrees of expression on the tumor cell plasma membrane.

Dynamics of inclusion of immunodominance are permissive redistribution as recharacterized indices for further potential increases of epitope expression to T lymphocytes. Recombinant tumor-specific proteins are currently among the most promising candidate anticancer vaccines, and monitoring of cancer vaccine trials should systemically include the assessment of HLA association with responsiveness [12].

Complex nature dynamics of the dominance of antigen presentation is hence a consideration of vital significance in turnover processing of particularly antigen presenting cells in general terms. Distribution preference dynamics are prominent mechanisms within the profile specificity of indices of activation of T lymphocytes.

MHC class I expression is up regulating during progression and therapy of HPV16-associated tutors and this may have important implications in the development of immunotherapeutic strategies [13]. Realization of system profiles of antigenicity are hence a complex integrative interplay of molecular dominance as determined by the evolutionary exposure of epitopes within the further development of sequence specificity of T cell receptor.

T Cell Specific Receptor

Lymphocyte specific antigen receptor is hence a process of selectivity in terms of antigenicity phenomena as expressed within the profile dynamics of redistribution of given antigen moieties as expressed on the lymphocyte/antigen presenting cells on the cell plasma membrane. Immunodominance redefines the quantitative affinity of receptivity of T lymphocytes as terms of pressure dynamics of redistributed membrane epitopes.

With regard to such immune defined pressure dynamics, the fluidity of the cell membrane may encompass the T lymphocyte specific receptor in terms that include the realization of binding affinity of the groove molecular structure of the MHC bearing cells. The status of the immune system in timor-bearing animal is capable of defining the MHC profile of the tutor cells; MHC class I-negative metastatic colonies are generated in immunocompetent animals, and MHC class I-positive colonies in T cell deficient individuals [14]. The production of incremental expressivity of such binding is itself dictated as gain/loss dimensions of surface antigen as expressed by tumor cells that in turn enhances the properties of biologic activation of the immune cells and of the antigen presenting cells. Tumor neoantigen heterogeneity thresholds provide a time window for combination immunotherapy where checkpoint blockade immunotherapy can become more effective [15]. Specificity issues allow for permissive interplay as possessed by and further enhanced by the antigen moiety interactivity with the antigen presenting cells. Such conditions provide general and specific attributes to immunodominant epitopes in general.

Conclusion

Bypass phenomena of direct and indirect cross-reacting antigen presentation are integral to systems of potentiality that are significantly dependent on pathways of molecular interplay as defining receptivity and epitope presentation. It is with regard to system profiles of immunity that the reactivity of T lymphocytes both dimensionalizes the attributes of antigen dominance and also of potent interactivity of the MHC molecule as dictated by antigen/receptor binding. The close semblance theme with regard to profile shifts in epitope expression allow for a significant degree of interplay that is itself self-potentiating.

REFERENCES

[1] Friedman J, Moore EC, Zolkind P, Robbins Y, Clavijo P, Sun L "Neoadjuvant PD-1 immune checkpoint blockade reverses functional immunodominance among tumor antigen-specific T cells" *Clin Cancer Res* 2020;26(3):679-689.

[2] Schreiber H, Wu TH, Nachman J, Fast WM "Immunodominance and tumor escape" *Semin Cancer Biol* 2002;12(1):25-31.

[3] Sahin U, Tureci O "Personalized vaccines for cancer immunotherapy" *Science* 2018;359(6382):1355-1360.

[4] Kreiter S, Vormehr M, de Roemer N, Diken M, Lower M, Diekmann J et al. "Mutant MHC class II epitopes drive therapeutic immune responses to cancer" *Nature* 2015;520(7549):692-6.

[5] Tran E, Ahmadzadeh M, Lu YC, Gros A, Turcotte S, Robbins PF et al. "Immunogenicity of somatic mutations in gastrointestinal cancers" *Science* 2015;350(6266):1387-90.

[6] Choi J, Meilleur CE, Mansour Haeryfar SM "Tailoring in vivo cytotoxicity assays to study immunodominance in timor-specific CD8+ T cell responses" *J Vis Exp* 2019;(147)dpo"1-3791/59531.

[7] Bhatia R, Gaitam SK, Cannon A, Thompson C, Hall BR, Aithal A et al. "Cancer-associated mucins: role in immune modulation and metastasis" *Cancer Metastasis Rev* 2019;38(1-2):334-236.

[8] Zamora AE, Crawford JC, Allen EK, Guo XZ, Bakke J, Carter RA et al. "Pediatric patients with acute lymphoblastic leukaemia generate abundant and functional neoantigen-specific CD8+ T cell responses" *Sci Transl Med* 2019;11(498):eaat8549.

[9] Flecken T, Schmidt N, Hild S, Gostick E, Drognitz O, Zeiser R et al. "Immunodominance and functional alterations of timor-associated antigen-specific CD8+ T cell responses in hepatocellular carcinoma" *Hepatology* 2014;59(4):1415-26.

[10] Svane IM, Engel AM "Immune selection in murine tumors. Ph.d thesis" *APMIS suppl* 2003;(106):1-46.

[11] Garcia-Lora A, Algarra I, Garrido F "MHC class I antigens, immune surveillance, and tutor immune escape" *J Cell Physiol* 2003;195(3):346-55.

[12] Bioley G, Guillaume P, Luescher I, Yeh A, Dupont B, Bhardwaj N et al. "HLA- class I -associated immunodominance affects CTL responsiveness to an ESO recombinant protein tumor antigen vaccine" *Clin Cancer Res* 2009;15(1):299-306.

[13] Mikyskova R, Bubenik J, Vonka V, Smahel M, Indrova M, Bieblova J et al. "Immune escape phenotype of HPV16-associated tumors: MHC class I expression changes during progression and therapy" *Int J Oncol* 2005;26(2):521-7.

[14] Algarra I, Garcia-Lora A, Cabrera T, Ruiz-Cabello F, Garrido F "The selection of tutor variants with altered expression of classical and nonclassical MHC class I molecules: implications for tumor immune escape" *Cancer Immunol Immunother* 2004;53(10):904-10.

[15] Aguade-Gorgorio G, Sole R "Tumour neoantigen heterogeneity thresholds provide a time window for combination immunotherapy" *JR Soc Interface* 2020;17(171):20200736.

Chapter 9

SYSTEMS OF UNSTABLE IMMUNODOMINANCE OF ANTIGEN AS FORMULAS FOR CENTRAL IMMUNOSUPPRESSION IN TUMOR CELL EXPANSION

ABSTRACT

The variabilities of instability of the antigenic profiles of growing, proliferating and spreading tumor cells allow for the significance of an immunosuppression that drives specifically the tumor biology of a given lesion. It is in terms that are highly specific for a central immunosuppression phenomenon that participating formulas are profile identity for further spread as the primary lesion initiates and further propagates expansion of whole subsets of tumor cells. The density quantitation realizations of the carcinogenesis induces a participating codominance as dictated by systems of unstable antigenicity on the surface of groups of tumor cells.

Introduction

The distributional pressure immune density of epitopes on tumor cells is paramount consideration within a heterogeneous tumor antigen dominance. The development of novel protocols for the induction of tolerance and new approaches to immunomodulation has been facilitated by advances in HLA technology [1]. In such terms, the quantitative presence of antigen associated with tumor biology conclusively dominates the performance of adoptively transferred immunotherapy as dictated by systems of redistribution of such antigen. Mucin-associated sialyl-Tn (sTn) antigens bind to receptors on dendritic cells, macrophages and natural killer cells resulting in overall immunosuppression by either receptor masking or inhibition of cytolytic activity [2]. The revocable presence of tumor associated antigen as demonstrably indicated by the prototype melanoma model indicates the possible realization of tumor antigenicity as performed by ex vivo expansion of tumor infiltrating lymphocytes or of antigen specific cytotoxic T lymphocytes.

Tumor Dynamics

Paramount presence and persistence of TAA within a dynamic population of dynamically turnover lesions are performance attributes that highly characterize tumors in general as indicated by the metastases that are variably and also specifically variant reproductions of the original neoplastic lesion.

In such terms, evolving dimensions clearly indicate instability of the Tumor Associated Antigens (TAA) as significant participation within systems of oligoclonal reproduction of cytotoxic T lymphocytes (CTL) and tumor infiltrating lymphocytes (TIL). Impaired anti-cancer immunity can be attributed to loss of immunodominant epitopes, down regulated major histocompatibility complex, and immunosuppressive microenvironment and also aberrant negative co-stimulatory signals [3]. It is significant to consider the dominance of a given antigen within a tumor cell population as simple factual and primal performance parameters that specifically evade the immunosurveillance of the body system. Immunodominance deters the response to other tumor antigens thereby favoring escape [4]. Terms that reproducibly promote systems of reactivity and of tumor regression indicate the probable participation of tumor growth and proliferation within the system pathway modulation of inherent tumor cell turnover.

ANTIGENICITY

Participation phenomena promote system shared antigenicity within the realization spherical modulatory pathways of antigen associated with pronounced immune suppression that in turn centrally induce tolerance as the tumor cell individually grows, proliferates and spreads. Current approaches to cancer immunotherapy provides new examples of epitope mimicry between cancer antigens and normal tissue antigens [5].

In terms derivative of any dimensions of reproducibility or of stable applicability to immune response, it is clear to consider promotional events as themselves unstable participants in the metastases phenomenon. It is within the conceptual creativity phenomenon of tumor biology that the systems of immune surveillance further confront the distributional density of epitopes as dictated by turnover of lymphocyte sets and subsets.

IMMUNOSURVEILLANCE

Promotional considerations point to a predominance of import distribution of TAA that confronts the immune responsiveness to the tumor that primarily dis coordinates the immunosurveillance as pathway modulatory subsets. It is within the instability of tumor cell biologic pathways that the further immunity response to the lesion proves permissive in terms of identity immune antigenicity and of a fundamentally plastic adaptability phenomenon. It is simply the realization of such adaptability that immunosurveillance phenomena both promote and further modulate tumor cell plasticity as central immunosuppression. The confrontational considerations of such adaptability allow for multiple forms of evasion as conclusive phenomena of the immune evasion. The identity formulations of tumor antigenicity indicate the further substantial derivation of tumor cells that specifically spread as terms of derivation of immunosuppression. The concomitant formulation of tumor evasive dimensions indicates the loss of antigenicity as driver dominance in turnover modulation.

The immune system is thus rendered centrally suppressed within the system profiles of an immunity reactive redirection. Immunotherapeutic concepts in neurooncology have mainly been hampered by poor definition of relevant antigens and selective measures to target the central nervous system [6]. The immune response is adopted within participating formulas driving the tumor cell growth, proliferation and spread as dictated by such evasive patterns of response by the tumor cells. It is further to be realized that the systems of protection against cancer cells are modulated forms of adaptation of the immune response to central immunosuppression. Immunoediting and immunodominance are the premier setbacks in peptide-based vaccine against cancer [7].

Reformulations

Repetitive reformulations of antigenicity identity are therefore a cardinal participation within systems of immune response directly driven by the involvement of lymphocyte subsets borne out by the promotional characters of the antigenicity. System pathway derivation is conclusive demonstration within the heterogeneity of a neoplastic group of subset modulation within the tumor cell pathway delineations. The distributional participation of an injury is identifiable system promotion of predominance of the antigen. The participation formulas allow for modulation in terms of induction phenomena of a quasi strict and continuous participation of the central immunosuppression formulations.

The further characteristics of such participations are permissive in terms of plasticity of response of the immune system as a whole. Immune selective pressure occurring during cancer immunoediting shapes tutor features; however in the "escape" phase, the tutor itself has the chance to influence the immunologic response [8]. It is the co-predominance of such participation that the formulas for response are inherent adaptability of the specific reformulations of tumor growth, proliferation and spread. Tumor endothelial marker 1-specific DNA vaccination targets tutor vasculature and this has therapeutic potential [9].

The overall significance of tumor cell turnover are hence the dominance attributes of an injury that is primarily adaptive within the formulas for further expansion and spread of the tumor lesion. It is within system profiles as adaptability that the realization of the carcinogenic origin of the lesion further participates within the promotional facilitation of such injury in terms of immune evasion.

FACILITATION

The promotional facilitation of immune evasions of the tumor cells is a modulation that specifically conforms the immunosuppression within systems for further change in immunity identity and in quantification immune antigenicity. The simplification of such central immunosuppression points towards formulas as dictated by an antigenicity beyond epitope participation. Discovery of immune checkpoint inhibitors in particular have validated immune cells as potential players for effective cancer treatment [10].

The redistributional biology of system pathways of immune evasion further participates as inductional nature of the tumor antigenicity. The formulas for such distinction allow for the emergence of integers for further change in immune response. The derivational participation of the carcinogenic event is injurious to an immune response that primarily evades the dominance attributes of specific forms of tumor cell antigenicity. In such terms the emergence of attributes of conformity are permissive for a primary event in immune evasion.

Conclusion

The modulation of tumor cell antigenicity is a primary induction of formulas of confrontation that are derived from participating factions of promotional plasticity, a plasticity that is strictly and specifically driven by forceful conformation of a central immunosuppression driven by attributes of simple antigen density on the surface of groups and subgroups of tumor cells.

It is as evidential formulas of participation that the overall significance of carcinogenic injury identifies the antigen dominance as itself derived from adaptive biology of the immune response itself. The further significance of such immune response adaptation is driver specific and dominates the formulas for further participation of the central immunosuppression induced also by the tumor cells.

References

[1] Montgomery RA, Tatapudi VS, Leffell MS, Zachary AA "HLA in transplantation" *Nat Rev Nephrol* 2018;14(9):558-570.

[2] Bhatia R, Gautam SK, Cannon A, Thompson C, Hall BR, Aithal A et al. "Cancer-associated mucins: role in immune modulation and metastasis" *Cancer Metastasis Rev* 2019;38(1-2):223-236.

[3] Li A, Yi M, Qin S, Chu Q, Luo S, Wu K "Prospects for combining immune checkpoint blockade with PARP inhibition" *J Hematol Oncol* 2019;12(1):98.

[4] van Waes C, Monach PA, Urban JL, Wortzel RD, Schreiber H " Immunodominance deters the response to other tumor antigens

thereby favouring escape: prevention by vaccination with tumor variants elected with cloned cytolytic T cells in vitro" *Tissue Antigens* 1996;47(5):399-407.

[5] Rose NR "Negative selection, epitope mimicry and autoimmunity" *Curr Opin Immunol* 2017;49:51-55.

[6] Platten M, Bunse L, Wick W, Bunse T "Concepts in glioma immunotherapy" *Cancer Immune Immunother* 2016;65(10):1269-75.

[7] Myc LA, Gamian A, Myc A "Cancer vaccines. Any future?" *Arch Immune Ther Exp* (Warsz) 2011;59(4):249-59.

[8] Merlo A, Dalla Santa S, Dolcetti R, Zanovello P, Rosato A "Reverse immunoediting: when immunity is edited by antigen" *Immune Lett* 2016;175"16-20.

[9] Facciponte JG, Ugel S, De Sanctis F, Li C, Wang L, Nair G et al. "Tumor endothelial marker 1-specific DNA vaccination targets tutor vasculature" *J Clin Invest* 2014;124(4):1497-511.

[10] Kumai T, Fan A, Harabuchi Y, Celis E "Cancer immunotherapy: moving forward with peptide T cell vaccines" *Curr Opin Immune* 2017;47:57-63.

Chapter 10

FAILED IMMUNOSURVEILLANCE AS FAILED DENDRITIC CELL ANTIGEN PRESENTATION—SUBSTITUTION OF SPECIFIC TUMOR ANTIGENICITY BY DIFFERENTIATION ASSOCIATED ANTIGENICITY

ABSTRACT

The dynamics of turnover of immune system pathways are ongoing pathways of active and also, to a lesser extent, passive procedural mechanics in antigen presentation. The integral projection of such mechanics is derivative increment in a failed activation series of steps in decontrol of homeostatic mechanisms inherent to immunosurveillance in the initial steps of attempted immune response. Such considerations allow for active participation of heterogeneous mechanisms within simple dynamics of turnover of T lymphocytes as determined by considered suppression of component immune response. It appears that specific and unique antigenicity is substituted for common differentiation or tumor-associated antigenicity widespread in many other tissues of the body.

INTRODUCTION

Attempts at manipulating the immunogenicity of given tumors have indicated the central roles played by the cellular pathways of the immune system. Results indicate that synthetic vaccine development is amenable to structure-activity relationship studies for optimisation of carbohydrate-based cancer vaccines [1]. It is interesting and vital to consider activation of T lymphocytes as projected by potentiating antibodies and cytokines as primary mechanisms in such immunogenicity promotion. The inability of melanoma patients to mount an effective antitumor response and the distinction between antigenicity (to express a tumor antigen) and immunogenicity (to elicit an effective antitumor response) is essential [2]. In terms of an overall series of dimensions, the unique attributes of antitumor immune responses are paramount considerations in attempted elucidation of immunogenicity enhancement. Cell morphogenesis and tumorigenesis are associated with changes in the glycoprotein profiles of the outer cell membranes [3]. The development of molecular techniques have allowed the study of activation steps of tumor infiltrating lymphocytes both quantitatively and qualitatively in the understanding the molecular nature of tumor antigenicity.

TUMORIGENESIS

The emergence of various tumors in patients on certain immunosuppressive agents such as azathioprine and cyclosporine in transplant patients, or in patients with congenital immunodeficiency syndromes, indicate a critical series of roles played by specific mechanisms of immunosurveillance in general and specific terms. Differences in the expression levels of tumor-associated antigens in cancers contrasted with normal cells (such as heat shock proteins, alpha-fetoprotein and carcino-embryonic antigen) are potential antitumor targets [4]. In such contexts the initial stages of such immunosurveillance are highly critical processes in immune mechanistic attempts at tumor control. Mapping the tumor immunopeptidome by mass spectrometry comprehensively accounts for the pathophysiologically relevant antigenic signature of human malignancies [5]. In the development of a full exposition of such concepts, the emergence of selectivity within the immune responses to tumors involves the defining terms of dysfunctionality of T cell responses involving both CD4+ and CD8+ cytotoxic cells. In terms of a full repertoire of modeled interactivities it has become obvious to consider the centrality of antigen-presenting cells in the evolving antitumor response of the immune system.

The distributive potentiality of immunogenicity is fundamental to the T cells in general response to both differentiation antigens and unique tumor antigens in initial immunosurveillance processes. Tumor-Associated carbohydrate antigens that define tumor malignancy as a basis for development of anti-cancer vaccines [6]. It is the evolution of such immunosurveillance that redefines the whole integral series of manoeuvres in the immunogenicity potentiation. The further development of the immune responses to tumors allows the emergence and development of immunogenicity of specific tumor antigens. Due to the low immunogenicity of tumor-associated carbohydrate antigens, a powerful carrier system is required to enhance immune responses; virus-like particles are a promising platform for delivering such tumor-associated carbohydrate antigens to the immune system [7].

POOR ANTIGENICITY

Subversive attributes of poor antigenicity or of nonexpression of antigenicity by several tumors are poorly understood. The simple nonrecognition by the immune system of tumor specific antigens in specific reference to differentiation antigens is closely linked to the widespread expression of such differentiation antigens in normal tissues in general. Hence, there exists a preferential series of roles as recognized activation antigen molecules of such nonspecific differentiation antigens in the further evolution of the failed immunosurveillance of tumors in general.

In such terms, the re-characterization of recognition mechanisms by cellular immunogenicity is integral to the simultaneous activation of the immune effector cells against tumors. Encapsulation of tumor-assocated antigens in polymer nanoparticles is a potential approach to increase efficiency of antigen deliver for antitumor vaccines [8].

Mechanistic properties of the antigen presentation cells such as professional dendritic cells appear a substantial attribute to the transformation of initial immunosurveillance stage to failed antitumor immunogenicity. In such terms, antigen presentation is integral failure to develop effective antitumor immune response. Neoplastic transformation is frequently associated with typical changes in the expression of sialyl Lewis(a) and sialyl Lewis(x) antigens and their adhesion to E-selectin and are carried by the carbohydrate chains of glycoproteins and glycolipids with adhesion to endothelium [9]. The evolution of such terms of reference is modeled on a series of dyshomeostatic pathways within the activation steps of both subsets of the T cell immune response. Such concept is referable to the dominant roles of differentiation antigens in such lymphocyte activation. It is relative to such failed T cell activation that professional antigen presentation cells acquire immunosuppressive attributes rather than robust immunogenic attributes.

Dynamics of Turnover of Lymphocytes

Dynamics of turnover of lymphocytes appear to account for the immunogenicity or failed immune response to tumors in general. In such terms, the nature of immune responses incorporate a redefinition of the initial immunosurveillance stage as evidenced failure of immunogenicity of tumor cells. The circumscribed models for activation of T cells are integral to dendritic cell biology as such. In specific terms non-recognition of antigens is a defining context within immunosurveillance pathways in the initial inception of the given tumor burden.

CD8+ T cells appear able to recognise tumor associated carbohydrate antigens in a conventional class I MHC-restricted fashion and Cytotoxic T Lymphocytes derived from normal donors respond with high efficiency to glycopeptides in vitro [10].

There appears to be a reciprocal relationship between normal transplantation antigens (H-2) and tumor-specific immunogenicity [11].

In various such contexts, the relative dynamics of increments in tumor growth redefine the evolving nature of progressive neoplasia as evidenced by the specific emergence of both evolving malignant transformation and spread of the neoplastic cells. In such terms, the conceptual recognition of tumor antigen non-recognition arises within the dyshomeostatic activation of both main subsets of T cell response.

CONTEXTUAL CONSIDERATIONS

The performance of experimental evidence as attributed to failed tumor antigenicity is hence the central consideration of current attempts to account for the antigen presentation steps as integral to T cell activation. The suppressive effect of tumor bearers' Lymph node cells is nonspecific and elicited also by bearers of an unrelated immunologically noncross-reacting methylcholanthrene-induced sarcoma [12]. The evolutionary course in such experiments point also to possible soluble cytokine actions within the further development of comparative immunosurveillance attempts in the context of failed antitumor antigenicity. The further determination of activation attempts of T cells is developmental biology of the differentiation effectiveness of such cells. In increasingly relevant distribution of such tumor evolution, it is significant to consider the reference terms of attributes of simple substitution pathways as evidenced by tumor progression. The component system pathways of lymphocyte activation are a further step in antigen presentation to such T cells as projected by MHC molecules referable to both class I and class II groups of antigen restriction presentation systems. It is relevant to such considerations that the burden of tumor cells is incremental within the substantial evolution of active suppressive mechanisms as borne out by the emergence of substitutive molecular mimicry of tumor-specific antigens.

Cell-mediated immune reactions may be probes of sensitisation to tumor-associated antigens of methylcholanthrene-induced mouse sarcomas [13].

Conclusion

Powerful modifying suppressive pathways as non-immunogenicity are central to understanding the basic mechanistic nature of an induced failed activation of the cellular immune responses to tumor cells. In such terms, the relative dimensions of incongruent antigenic presentation is evolving pathway central to the carcinogenesis process built within pathways of a failed immune response. The development of system models for such non-activation of T cells is evidential attribute within the natural evolution of a given tumor that is contextually progressive. The molecular nature of failed immune response arises as characterization of the immune system as a whole as integral terms of non-presentation of the tumor-specific antigens. The substituted differentiation antigens as widespread dynamics of failed antitumor immune response allows for the evolution of re-characterized neoplasia.

References

[1] Ingale S, Wolfert MA, Buskas T, Boons GJ "Increasing the antigenicity of synthetic timor-associated carbohydrate antigens by targeting Toll-like receptors" *Chembiochem* 2009;10(3):455-63.

[2] Gattoni-Celli S, Cole DJ "Melanoma-associated tumor antigens and their clinical relevance to immunotherapy" *Semin Oncol* 1996;23(6):754-8.

[3] Brocke C, Kunz H "Synthesis of tumor-associated glycopeptide antigens" *Bioorg Med Chem* 2002;10(10):3085-112.

[4] Liu CC, Yang H, Zhang R, Zhao JJ, Hao DJ "Tumor-associated antigens and their anti-cancer applications" *Eur J Cancer Care* (Engl) 2017;26(5):doi:10.1111.

[5] Freudenmann LK, Marcu A, Stevanovic S "Mapping the tutor human leukocyte antigen (HLA) ligandome by mass spectrometry" *Immunology* 2018;154(3):331-345,

[6] Hakomori S "Tumor-associated carbohydrate antigens defining tumor malignancy: basis for development of anti-cancer vaccines" *Adv Exp Med Biol* 2001;491:369-402.

[7] Sungsuwan S, Wu X, Huang X "Evaluation of virus-like particle-based tumor associated carbohydrate immunogen in a mouse tumor model" *Methods Enzymol* 2017;597:359-376.

[8] Spolbrig CM, Saucier-Sawyer JK, Cody V, Saltzman WM, Hanlon DJ "Polymer nanoparticles for immunotherapy from encapsulated timor-associated antigens and whole tumor cells" *Mol Pharm* 2007;4(1):47-57.

[9] Ugorski M, Laskowska A "Sialyl Lewis(a): a tumor-associated carbohydrate antigen involved in adhesion and metastatic potential of cancer cells" *Acta Biochim Pol* 2002P:49(2):303-11.

[10] Xu Y, Sette A, Sidney J, Gendler SJ, Franco A "Tumor-associated carbohydrate antigens: a possible avenue for cancer prevention" *Immunol Cell Biol* 2005;83(4):440-8.

[11] Haywood GR, McKhann "Antigenic specificities on murine sarcoma cells. Reciprocal relationship between normal transplantation antigens (H-2) and timor-specific immunogenicity" *J Exp Med* 1971;133(6):1171-87.

[12] Indrova M, Bubenik J "Inhibition of cell-mediated cytotoxicity against tumor-associated antigens by suppressor lymph node cells from mice bearing methylcholanthrene-induced sarcomas" *Neoplasma* 1979;26(4):405-12.

[13] Bubonic J, Indrova M, Malkovsky M, Simova J "Cell-mediated immune reactions as probes of sensitisation to timor-associated antigens of methylcholanthrene-induced mouse sarcomas" *Arch Geschuwulstforsch* 1981;51(4):349-53.

Chapter 11

PROJECTED RECEPTIVITY OF INTEGRAL GLIOMAS TO MALIGNANT TRANSFORMATION AS MODELED BY DYSFUNCTIONAL IMMUNOMODULATION

ABSTRACT

Conclusive participation of malignant transformation is integral to a receptivity phenomenon of involvement of system profiles that project beyond the conventional pathway formulas of such malignant transformation. It is further significant provocation of injury to glioma precursor cells that the overall models for transformation are specifically malignant in terms of the receptivity phenomena as borne out by the integral inclusion of carcinogenicity. The simple formulas as apparently projected by vascular endothelial cells are conformational attribute dysfunctionality of a receptivity of subsequent immune response of the glioma as malignant transformation.

INTRODUCTION

Immunomodulation of the immune homeostatic micro-environment is tentative manipulative series of measures in the control of suppressive action with regard to high grade gliomas. Lack of progress in treatment is due to essential infiltrativeness of the glioma, tumor protection by the blood-brain barrier, intrinsic resistance to induced cell death, and lack of dependence on single oncogenic pathways [1]. The concept of control of glioma cell antigenicity and proliferation are derivative inducing factors in the overall dimensional control with regard to antigen presentation and subsequent stimulation of the immuno modulation of such tumors. Understanding the intricate microenvironmental landscape will probably enhance the development of novel immunotherapy [2]. Inclusive phenomena induce a series of modulated dimensions in the altering of such processes as both MHC and non-MHC influences within a sphere of dynamic turnover within high grade gliomas.

The complex interactions within the substantial provoking environment of brain tumors in general allow for the emergence of further provoking influences as dictated especially by microglia and the important vascular antigens such as tenascin and intercellular adhesion molecule and vascular endothelial adhesion molecule. In such terms, overall induction constitutes potentially powerful stimulants of the immune system within the segregated environment as induced by the blood brain barrier.

DIMENSIONAL THEORY

Dimensional recovery of control of the immune response to tumor specific antigenicity is a complex interplay that enhances potentially the recovery of the systems of modulation of the immune responses set in operative attack to the glioma specific antigens. It is in such manner that exclusive phenomena of suppression of glioma cell biology is further confirmatory system of response on the part of microglia and astrocytes against systems of provoking response in immuno-modulation. A range of immunotherapeutic approaches include vaccines, checkpoint inhibitors, oncolytic viruses and gene therapies [3]. The reactivities of response go beyond simple modulated immune response but may participate within the responsive attributes of the cerebral vasculature of systems borne out by the turnover dynamics of blood flow on the one hand and a series of restituting immuno-modulation of glioma cell proliferation and spread. Due to the molecular heterogeneity, immuno-editing and profound immunosuppression, combinatorial approaches targeting multiple pathways tailored to the tutor genetic signature are required to induce effective therapy [4].

IMMUNOMODULATION

The suggestive responses of tumor infiltrating lymphocytes are indicative dimensions that dynamically and potentially inhibit tumor response to such cytokines as interferon gamma, Interleukin 1 and 6 and also adhesion molecules effective in vascular response to the growing glioma cells.

It is further to such conceptual system profiles that the ongoing emergence of glioma biologic indices further conform to distributional supply of cytokines that could suppress the interactive forces of increment in glioma growth. The simple attributes for persistence of immunomodulation are clearly conformational profile for re-distributional suppression of systems of receptivity and response as further attested by increments of glioma biologic actions. The unequivocal definition of glioma progression by conventional MRI remains difficult especially in the setting of immunotherapy induced by checkpoint inhibitors and dendritic cells [5].

PERMISSIVE DIMENSIONS

Provoking dimensions of immuno-modulation allow a permissive dimension in potential control of systems as projected by the overall specific antigenicities of a given glioma lesion within the spheres of control of response and potential tumor suppression. The implementation of immunotherapy via manipulative modulation of activation of cytotoxic T cells has hand an outstanding impact on peripheral cancers under certain clinical circumstances [6]. In such terms, the increments of response to tumor antigenicity are simple reference pathways of potential control of glioma biologic indices as further attested by the overall modulation as systems of strict response to glioma cell antigenicity.

In further conformation dimensions of suppressing response, the pathways of potentiality and of effective attributes of control of glioma growth attest to the overall non specificity reactivities as attested by active cytokine profiles for further potential control of glioma biology. Tumor-associated macrophages contribute to tutor growth and neovacularization and understanding of their roles in neovascularization of tutor is essential for future anti-angiogenic therapies [7]. Glioma-infiltrating myeloid cells including microglia comprise up to 30% of total tumor mass and may be involved in proliferation, motility survival and immunosuppression; acquired roles of an anti-inflammatory (M2) macrophage and microglial phenotype may suppress immune response [8].

CONSTITUTIVE RESPONSE

Deliberation of constitutive response that immunologically refashion the micro environment of glioma cells further attests to the substantial potential recovery of suppression formulas in the control of dynamic phenomena of tumor cell proliferation and spread. Immunotherapy with immune checkpoint inhibitors such as ipilimumab, nivolumab, and pembrolizumab provide clinical improvements in other advanced tutor for which conventional therapies have had limited success [9]. It is further to such responses that gliomas themselves are genetic models in their own right within systems of suppressive response as dictated by microglia and also to a lesser extent by astrocytes within the central nervous system.

The relative dimensions of immuno-stimulation and of immuno-modulation of the immune responses within a given glioma cell population are attested formulas that profile coordination systems for suppression of malignant transformation. Poor results in therapy may be due to the response of tumor-associated macrophages that create imbalances between innate and adaptive immunity and altered blood-brain barrier properties [10]. Novel neuro-oncology-specific concepts have refuted the classic dogma that the CNS is immuno-privileged and hence inaccessible to potent anti-tumor immunity [11]. Glioma cells interfere with anti-tumor immune responses by expressing immune inhibitory cell surface molecules such as HLA-G or by releasing soluble immunosuppressants such as transforming growth factor-beta [12]. In such terms the delivery of transforming factors within the segregated microenvironment conclusively denote reactive systems that arise specifically within units of response dictated by the vascular endothelium and also perivascular pericytes as directly controlled by vascular wall adhesion molecules.

PERFORMANCE DYNAMICS

The performance dimensions of dynamic interactions between glioma growth on the one hand, and the modulated immune response bespeak of active participation of malignancies that correlate with system profiles of glioma biologic actions. Vaccination, with or without dendritic cells, blockage of immune checkpoints and adoptive T cell transfer are mot studied in diffuse glioma immunotherapy [13].

In such manner, performance indices participate as conclusive phenomena of equilibrating influences of balanced equilibrium as borne out by antigenicity of the individual glioma cell. Mutant isocitrate dehydrogenase (IDH) is not only a disease-defining biomarker and oncogenic driver in glioma, but also a neoantigen and regulator of glioma immune evasion [14]. Mutations in the IDH1/2 genes are central to gliomagenesis in a high proportion of grade II and III gliomas and ongoing trials are examining vaccines against IDH1, small molecular inhibitors of IDH1 and IDH2 and, and metabolic components including NAD+ depletion to target IDH-mutated gliomas [15]. Integral participating influence is reflective dimension within equilibrating systems of receptivity that goes beyond response elements of the tumor transformation to malignancy. In such terms, the provoking redistribution of malignant injurious pathways are potentially simple caricatures of response that subserve receptivity profile dynamics.

CONCLUSION

It is further to dynamic turnover that gliomas, as integral indices of biologic receptivity, are both conformational profile models for the interpretative dynamics as borne out especially in terms of a malignant change within systems of vascular response. The profile participation of injury to the individual endothelial cell is further dimensional modeling of an injury that biologically provokes systems of receptivity in its own right.

In such terms, the performance indices are real antigenic participation within the vascular fields of receptivity of glioma precursor cells as confronted within the pathway evolutionary systems for such receptivity to carcinogenic stimuli. The apparent autonomies as portrayed by potential response elements include the further dimensions of receptivity that alternatively provoke response in terms of malignant transformation.

Projection profiles of such reactive receptivities conclusively participate as models of influence as attested by the performance of re-distributional dynamics of receptivity per se of the integral glioma lesion. It is significant to view the participation of receptivity to the overall vascular involvement in empowering malignant transformation within encompassed validity of response of such integral glioma response.

REFERENCES

[1] Lim M, Xia Y, Bettegowda C, Weller M "Current state of immunotherapy for glioblastoma" *Nat Rev Clin Oncol* 2018;15(7):422-442.

[2] Boussiotis VA, Charest A "Immunotherapies for malignant glioma" *Oncogene* 2018;37(9)"1121-1141.

[3] Lukas RV, Wainwright DA, Horbinski CM, Iwamoto FM, Sonabend AM "Immunotherapy against gliomas: is the breakthrough near?" *Drugs* 2019;79(17):1839-1848.

[4] Kamran N, Alghamri MS, Nunez FJ, Shah D, Asad AS, Candolfi M et al. "Current state and future prospects of immunotherapy for glioma" *Immunotherapy* 2018;10(4):317-339.

[5] Aquino D, Gioppo A, Finocchiaro G, Bruzzone MG, Cuccarini V "MRI in glioma immunotherapy: evidence, pitfalls, and perspectives" *J Immune Res* 2017;2017:5813951.

[6] Miyauchi JT, Tsirka S "Advances in immunotherapeutic research for glioma therapy" *J Neurol* 2018;265(4):741-756.

[7] Zhu C, Kros JM, Cheng C, Mustafa D "The contribution of timor-associated macrophages in glioma net-angiogenesis and implications for anti-angiogenic strategies" *Neuro Oncol* 2017;19(11):1435-1446.

[8] Arcuri C, Fioretti B, Bianchi R, Mecca C, Tubaro C, Beccari T et al. "Microglia-glioma cross-talk: a two way approach to new strategies against glioma" *Front Biosci* 2017;22:268-309.

[9] Preusser M, Lim M, Hafler DA, Reardon DA, Sampson JH "Prospects of immune checkpoint modulators in the treatment of glioblastoma" *Nat Rev Neural* 11(9):504-14.

[10] Vismara MFM, Donato A, Malara N, Presta I, Donato G "Immunotherapy in gliomas: are we reckoning without the innate immunity?" *Int J Immunopathol Pharmacy* 2019;33:20587384 19832278.

[11] Platten M, Bunse L, Wick W, Bunse T "Concepts in glioma immunotherapy" *Cancer Immunol Immunother* 2016;65(10):12690-75.

[12] Friese MA, Steinle A, Weller M "The innate immune response in the central nervous system and its role in glioma immune surveillance" *Onkologie* 2004;27(5):487-91.

[13] De Carli E, Delion M, Rousseau A "Immunotherapy in brain tumours" *Ann Pathol* 2017;37(1):117-126.

[14] Friedrich M, Bunse L, Wick W, Platten M "Perspectives of immunotherapy in iso citrate dehydrogenase-mutant gliomas" *Curr Opin Oncol* 2018;30(6):368-374.

[15] Chen R, Cohen AL, Colman H "Targeted therapeutics in patients with high-grade gliomas: past, present, and future" *Curr Treat Options* 2016;17(8):42.

Chapter 12

TUMOR CELL IDENTITY AS PROJECTED BY IMMUNOTOXINS WITHIN HETEROGENEITY AND HIERARCHICAL SYSTEMS OF PROGRESSION

ABSTRACT

The exponential systems of amplification of tumor cell infiltration and spread are related intimately to overall growth dimensions of a given brain tumor and as expounded within hemodynamics of supply to the parent lesion. The significant realization of spectra of susceptibility incorporate other performance indices as evidenced by systems of performance of the individual tumor cell within an induced milieu that exerts profound toxicity to dynamic turnover of the neoplasm. In such terms, the realization of cell infiltration and multiplication is a conjugate performance index of emerging systems of growth of such individual tumor cell and cells.

Introduction

The overall dimensions of immunotoxicity treatment of primary brain tumors and metastatic leptomeningeal neoplastic meningitis are well represented as targeted therapy for tumors. Convection-enhanced delivery of macromolecules is considered the leading delivery mode for the treatment of malignant gliomas [1]. The incremental involvement of such dimensions resolves also as terms of intra-tumoral distribution within such lesions as primary and recurrent malignant gliomas. Biologic intra-tumoral therapies are important due to their inherent potential to be both dynamically adaptive and target specific [2]. Immunotoxins are very promising as therapeutic tool for gliomas and human mesenchymal stem cells show tropism to tumor tissue [3]. The performance coordinates are further projected in terms of the potent toxic effects of such agents or conjugates that in turn bind to the cell surface receptors and are then transferred within the tumor cells. The incremental distribution of the immunotoxin is further qualified in terms of the overall dose of radio-reactivity rather than the concentration of these agents.

Simple extrapolation requires the consideration of tumor cell immunotoxicity as borne out by dynamics of turnover of the radio-immunotoxin in terms referable to the stability of this molecule.

Immunotoxins conjugated to targeting antibody or growth factors such as transferrin conjugate radio-toxicity include also consideration of the stability of the conjugate in the context also of stability of the tumor indices. Glycoprotein NMB is a transmembrane glycoprotein that is highly expressed in malignant gliomas and is thus an attractive target in tumor immunotherapy [4]. In such terms, the performance dynamics of intra-tumoral distribution is dependent on the mode of delivery of the agent such as would be noted in the context of intra-peritoneal, intravenous or intra-tumoral delivery.

In addition to inherent tumoricidal properties, immunotoxins stimulate secondary immune responses through T-cell activation; glioblastoma suppresses immune responses and this is a major hurdle to an effective immunomoxin-mediated antitumor response [5].

Radiotoxicity

The significance of tumor cell radio-toxicity is beset by the terms of reference of injury that significantly select the targeting susceptibility without the accompanying significant systemic toxicity. It should be realized that the delivery intra-thecally of immunotoxins is a model representation in the controlled systemic exposure to toxicity to cells such as normal brain tissue and other organs such as the liver that is richly endowed, for example, by transferrin receptors.

The further contributory range of influences of immunotoxins is corroborative evidence for the development of a profound toxic exposure of the tumor cells as illustrated by dimensions of incremental involvement of, particularly, primary brain tumors at time of diagnosis. A few promising therapies have emerged in the last decade and include biodegradable polymers for interstitial chemotherapy, convection-enhanced delivery of targeted toxins and locally injected genetically modified viruses [6]. The overall increments in toxic exposure of the neoplastic lesion allow for the evolution of immuno-therapy as stability dynamics homogenously or heterogeneously distributed within the tumor vascular supply. The resistance that develops intra-tumorally with conventional chemotherapy is significant within a milieu of ischemia; such ischemia induced resistance is not seen with the delivery of immuno-toxins which in turn involve problems of delivery to the bulk of the brain tumor. Convection-enhanced delivery generates pressure-driven flow that may potentially distribute drugs over large brain volumes [7].

Susceptibility Patterns

A biphasic redistribution delivery of some immuno-toxins such as transferrin conjugated to Cross Reacting Material is noted.

The profound sensitivity to diphtheria toxin in humans is further incorporated as tumor lesion creation as borne out by the overall dimensions of conjugate involvement, not only intra-cellularly, but also as extracellular ligation to cell surface receptors. The conformational identity of turnover of such cell surface receptors is prominent in terms of binding of the immunotoxin conjugate. The distribution intra-tumorally is reduced consequence to the actual binding to these receptors within significant punctate delivery and distribution within the lesion.

Performance-controlled inhibition further comprises the significant influence of tumor cell injury per se. In such terms, the emergency of injury to tumor cells is beset by terms of the heterogeneous nature of the brain tumor and as further compounded by an injury that excites further delivery within the lesion.

The most promising lines of investigative research in brain tumour therapy include non-cytotoxic drugs, immunotoxins, abiogenesis inhibitors and gene therapy [8]. Due to the increased expression of the transferrin receptor in brain gliomas, the successful delivery of anticancer agents to the tumor site and the capability to cross the blood brain barrier have indicated an important discovery [9].

The overall dimensions as significant stability dynamics of the immuno-conjugate are relative indices for suppression of tumor cell susceptibility to the parent protein core that constitutes the toxic moiety. The incremental differences in distribution are paramount considerations within simple hemodynamic reappraisal as borne out by such heterogeneous lesions as glioblastoma.

Compound Influence

Turnover indices of necrosis of tumor cells exposed to immunotoxins are derivative mesenchymal elements and vascularity components within the brain tumor. The significant performance redistribution of injury is compounded by the realization of susceptibility dynamics. The overall incremental exposure to such lesions as bulk-resected tumors at surgery is directed optimally to residual foci of the neoplasm. The scope of penetration within systems of cellular infiltration and cell division is incorporated as evidential reconstitution of the performance dynamics of tumor cell susceptibility. A direct correlation exists between levels of Interleukin-13 Receptor mRNA expression and poor patient prognosis; immunosuppressive genes related to IL-13Ralpha2 may play a role in glioblastoma progression [10].

Conclusion

The realization of injury to toxicity phenomena response are significant as terms or incremental development of the injury that is exerted in the presence of a near-intact blood brain barrier as well expounded by turnover integers and as further evidenced by decreased tumor mass seen by in vivo imaging and prolongation of patient survival. The further conformational dimensions of the neoplastic lesion are paramount considerations in terms of such performance indices as intra-tumoral distribution of the immuno-conjugate. The identity of such sustained toxicity is evidenced by the exposure to toxic protein that specifically and necessarily incriminates the overall targeting of the single tumor cell. The buildup exponential increments in immunotoxin redistribution within the tumor lesion are performance-permissive in terms that realize susceptibility spectra as exhibited within the infiltrative margins of the parent lesion.

The hierarchical exponents of realization of immunotoxin exposure of brain tumors is operative dimension that includes dynamics of turnover of the immuno-conjugate as evidenced by systems of performance indices of tumor cell infiltration and spread within the central nervous system.

Substantial evidence indicates that if appropriately re-directed, T cells can precisely eradicate neoplasms; a fully human bispecific antibody (hEGFRvIII-CD3 bi-scFv) redirects human T cells to use gliomas expressing a tumor-specific mutation of the EGFR (EGFRvIII) [11].

The overall conformations of redistribution do not only involve permeability of an intact blood brain barrier but also the tumoral dynamics of neoplastic cell turnover per se. In such terms, the emergence of cellular targeting is further dimensional index as evidenced by immuno-conjugates that incorporate selective receptor binding.

Perpetuation of sustained immunotoxicity is viable option within the significant heterogeneity of brain tumors with the realization of injury conforming to the infiltrative behavior of such lesions. The emergence of trajectorial dimensions of exponential growth and spread of the neoplasms is significant also as sustained growth of the parent lesion per se. The inclusive hemodynamics are integrative within the conformational geometry of a lesion that is continuously evolving and re-dimensionalizing within systems of performance identity and projection.

References

[1] Vandergrift WA, Patel SJ, Nicholas JS, Varma AK "Convection-enhanced delivery of immunotoxins and radioisotopes for treatment of malignant gliomas" *Neurosurg Focus* 2006;20(4):E13.

[2] Loya J, Zhang C, Cox E, Achrol AS, Kesari S "Biological intratumoral therapy for the high-grade glioma part I: intratumoral delivery and immunotoxins" *CNS Oncol* 2019;8(3):CNS38.

[3] Zhang Y, Sun X, Huang M, Ke Y, Wang J, Liu X "A novel bispecific immunomoxin delivered by human bone marrow-derived mesenchymal stem cells to target blood vessels and vasculogenic mimicry of malignant gliomas" *Drug Des Devel There* 2015;9:2947-59.

[4] Kuan CT, Wakiya K, Keir ST, Li J, Herndon JE 2nd, Pastan I et al. "Affinity-matured anti-glycoprotein NMB recombinant immunotoxins targeting malignant gliomas and melanomas" *Int J Cancer* 2011;129(1):111-21.

[5] Chandramohan V, Bao X, Yu X, Parker S, McDowall C, Yu YR et al. "Improved efficacy against malignant brain tumours with EGFRwt/EGFRvIII targeting immunomoxin and checkpoint inhibitor combinations" *J Immunother Cancer* 2019;7(1):142.

[6] Rain NG, Soling A, Heidecke V "Novel therapies for malignant gliomas: a local affair?" *Neurosurg Focus* 2006;20(4):E9.

[7] Buonerba C, Di Lorenzo G, Marinelli A, Federico P, Palmieri G, Imbimbo M et al. "A comprehensive outlook on intracerebral therapy of malignant gliomas" *Crit Rev Oncol Hematol* 2011;80(1):54-68.

[8] Basso U, Armani M, Vastola F, Brandes AA "Non-ctotoxic therapies for malignant gliomas" *J Neurooncolo* 2002;58(1):57-69.

[9] Tortorella S, Karagiannis TC "Transferrin receptor-mediated endocytosis: a useful target for cancer therapy" *J Membr Bio* 2014;247(4):291-307L

[10] Han J, Puri RK "Analysis of the cancer genome atlas (TCGA) database identifies an inverse relationship between interleukin-13 receptor alpha1 and alpha2 gene expression and poor prognosis and drug resistance in subjects with glioblastoma multiforme" *J Neurooncol* 2018;136(3):463-474.

[11] Gideon PC, Schaller TH, Chitneni SK, Choi BD, Kuan CT, Suryadevara CM et al. "A rationally designed fully human EGFRvIII:CD3-Targeted bispecific antibody redirects human T cells to treat patient-derived intracerebral malignant glioma" *Clin Cancer Res* 2018;24(15):3611-3631.

Chapter 13

DIMENSIONS OF REPRODUCIBLE MALIGNANT TRANSFORMATION AS BRAIN INFILTRATION BY GLIOMA

ABSTRACT

Frameworks of operability and dysregulation are paramount considerations in the evolutionary history of a malignant glioma in particular as further emphasized by the embryonic nature of characterization of the cells of origin of a given neoplasm. It is in terms of evolving constitution that the infiltrated surrounding brain tissue of a malignant glioma recapitulates the derivative nature of oncogenesis with its multi-varied dimensions of spread into the surrounding tissues as support and inducing influence in oncogenesis. Radio-nuclides are parametric models that attempt directing suppression primarily of such infiltrative margins of malignant gliomas, as well exemplified by models of generation and duplication of the malignant transformation process from the initial stage of conception to the culmination as infiltrative margins of a given malignant glioma.

Introduction

The conceptual approach of treating malignant gliomas with radio-labeled antibodies is based on the tumor directed toxicity of the radio-isotope within frameworks of attempted concentrating localization to the tumor as directed by systems of operative and also external radiation. Neoadjuvant nivolumab in glioblastoma patients resulted in enhanced expression of chemokine transcripts, higher immune cell infiltration and augmented TCR clonal diversity among timor-infiltrating T lymphocytes, indicating a local immunomodulatory effect of PD-1 blockade [1]. The significance of such attempts is within the scope of realization as borne out by schemes of operative management of newly diagnosed patients as well as for recurrent tumor patients. The anti-cancer effects of dietary phytochemical such as curcumin can promote targeting of multiple signaling pathways in glioblastoma [2]. Within such scenarios, the further participation of injury pharmacokinetics directed mainly towards the tumor mass is dependent on several hemodynamic parameters as borne out by such measures as hyperthermia that both increases tumor blood supply and also vascular permeability.

Radio Labeling

The further improved radio -labeling isotopes and the specific attached antibody affinities are attempts within the system profiles of the degree of stability of both radio-nuclides and the antibody conjugates.

The lack of functional dendritic cells from the brain causes the brain to lack the priming of systemic immune responses to glioma antigens [3].

As such, the further involvement of the targeting dynamics approaches a specific enhancement as demonstrable within such therapeutic attempts. Challenges of brain cancer therapy clinically are to overcome chemo- and radio-resistance, to improve drug deliver to tumors and the development of effective drug screening [4]. The significant formulation of essential dynamics are proof of principle within systems that operate in vivo as terms of reference and as formatting pathways of decreased viability of the relevant tumor cells within encompassed tumor integrity.

Labelling with the alpha particle emitting Bi-213 is promising due to the high linear energy transfer and the very short tissue range; future development needs to focus on improvement of the stability of the compound and application of dedicated catheter systems to improve intra-tumoral distribution within infiltrative margins of the glioma [5]. Performance attributes allows the creation of permissive elements within the significant infiltrating potentialities of malignant gliomas in particular. The administration of radionuclides-labeled monoclonal antibodies is severely compromised by the systemic toxicity patterns particularly to normal neural tissues and to the bone marrow. As such, the specific modes of administration has been further explored in terms of incremental escalating doses of the targeting antibody conjugate as dictated by non-systemic routes of delivery.

The significant selectivity that has been developed is compartmental in mode of administration as performed especially into tumor cavities either as spontaneous cysts or as post surgical resection cavities.

Stabilized Tumor Dynamics

Stabilization of the tumor dynamics by such delivered radio-nuclides is an observed phenomenon within the performance of delivery parameters as borne out also by delayed recurrence of the tumors and at times by prolongation of survival of the tumor animal models especially xenograft rat human systems. Results from single agent targeted therapy trials have been modest; lack of efficacy result from poor blood brain barrier penetration, the genetic heterogeneity of the tumors and the development of resistance mechanisms [6]. Participation of tumor cell injury is correlated with a concentrated localization of such radio-nuclides that emit either alpha or beta radio-emission. A multi-disciplinary approach to the therapy of glioma and glioblastoma is indicated [7]. It is further to such approaches that the targeting of tumor cells is problematic in the abnormal brain tissue invaded by the expanding and infiltrative advancing edge of malignant gliomas.

Long noncoding RNAs show increasing aberrant expression in glioma tissues and cell lines and may be critical for glioma initiation, progression and malignant phenotype; IncRNAs are potential biomarkers and therapeutic targets in gliomas [8].

Tumor-associated macrophages are significant in contributing to tumor growth, metastasis and neovascularization; potential therapeutic targets to intervene in tumor angiogenesis are being explored [9].

Brain Infiltration

It is further to such considerations that the brain tissue infiltrated by the growing edge of malignant neoplasms but especially by malignant gliomas is inherently abnormal and reproduces a micro-environment that is strongly conducive to the further growth and spread of the tumor.

Molecular networks govern glioma biology and focus on intracellular signaling molecules in gliomas that associate with each other and regulate refractoriness against current therapy [10].

The paradoxical systems conducive to further spread of a malignant glioma including the glioblastoma are paramount considerations in the therapeutic approach to the tumor with the added considerations of spread as dysfunctional conditioning of the parent neoplasms. The vasculature of neoplasms is an expression of such a concept of infiltrated brain tissue in supplying the essential milieu for tumor growth and spread. In such terms, mesenchymal vascular support for neoplasms enhances and further provokes the gliomagenesis and directs in multi-varied ways the development of essential support for the parent tumor and infiltrating edge of the glioma.

MALIGNANT TRANSFORMATION

Such considerations revolve in terms of the nature of the infiltrated brain tissue within encompassed definition of regions for malignant transformation. Recent research has proposed canonical transient receptor potential channels to be newly emerged potential drug targets for glioma and are involved in proliferation, migration, invasion, angiogenesis and metabolism of glioma cells [11]. The actual process of origin of the infiltrating gliomatous cells is derivative exponent of the surrounding brain tissue in terms of incremental employment of such derived trophic factor supply and angiogenesis. The Cancer Genome Atlas and other projects have shown the somatic alterations and molecular subtypes of glioma at diagnosis; however, gliomas develop along significant cellular and molecular evolutionary courses during disease progression [12]. It is indeed the nature of transformations occurring within the adjacent surrounding brain tissue that there arises incremental growth and recurrence of neoplasms as so well exemplified by microscopic foci of recurrent glioma left viable at surgery. The terms of reference of such infiltrative phenomena include the establishment of amplification of trophic effect and above all of transforming potentiality within systems of modeled gene transduction and protein translation and also within the inherent production of such mediators as adhesion molecules. Multi-targeted kinase inhibitors or combinations of agents targeting different mitogenic pathways may overcome the resistance of tumors to single agent targeted therapies [13].

Such systems that are applicable to gliomas are relevant with similar emphasis to malignant neoplasms as a whole and offer formidable hurdles to the complete expiration of a given malignant neoplasm. It is further to supporting frameworks of the tumor that the incremental distinctive and advancing nature of infiltrative phenomena in the primary neoplasm is itself subject to the nature of the infiltrating edges of tumor cells and that these latter are patterned by the surrounding infiltrated brain tissue. It is still a struggle to develop modalities to expose the entire tumor to therapeutics at pharmacologically meaningful quantities [14].

Conclusion

The paradoxical attributes of exposing influences to the infiltrating margins of a given malignant glioma are testimonial parameters within encompassed micro-environmental factors of influence that beget the malignant transformation as genitor event in oncogenesis. The distributional nature of the primary neoplasm and its genesis includes derivative phenomena that reproduce the essential requirements of the original cell changes in oncogenesis and neogenesis of the parent neoplasm. Pathway inhibition, via multi-site kinase inhibitors or a carefully selected combination of molecular drugs with or without cytotoxic agents, is currently being evaluated in clinical trials [15].

In such terms, the overall configurational dimensions of incremental effect are expression of the amplifying nature of the malignant transformation events within systems for further growth and spread of initial oncogenesis steps. It is further to this that the parameters of control and loss of control in cell division and spread are amplification in essential nature and further conform to necessities of induction within embryonic terms of reference in oncogenesis and gliomagenesis. Epidermal growth factor receptor is commonly amplified and/or mutated in high-grade gliomas; the ability of certain neoplastic cells to maintain signaling through AKT and ERK under EGFR inhibition may constitute a potential mechanism of resistance by tumor cells to escape the anti-proliferative activity of EGFR inhibitors [16].

Parametric redefinition of such processes is fundamental to a realization of cell injury in a manner that is of importance in considering the toxicity spectra of induced action when delivering radionuclides labeled with targeting monoclonal antibodies. It is indeed in redefined conceptual approaches that the glioma and neoplasms in general both derive the incremental nature of neoplastic progression. Consequential attributes of redefined tumor parameters conclusively model patterns of derivation as substituted indices of biologic progression of a given glioma. Further reproductive patterns of pattern duplication require a modification in molecular frameworks in the employment of toxic injuries inflicted to tumor cells and exclusively to such tumor cells. Such considerations are particularly applicable to targeted therapies to gliomas that primarily infiltrate and subsequently and secondarily undergo cell division.

References

[1] Schaper KA, Rodriguez-Ruiz ME, Diez-Valle R, Lopez-Janeiro A, Porciuncula A, Idolate MA et al. "Neoadjuvant Nivolumab modifies the tumor immune microenvironment in resectable glioblastoma" *Nat Med* 2019;25(3):470-476.

[2] Shahcheraghi SH, Zangui M, Lotfi M, Ghayour-Mobarhan M, Ghorbani A, Jaliani HZ et al. "Therapeutic potential of cur cumin in the treatment of glioblastoma multiforme" *Crr Pharm Des* 2019;25(3):333-342.

[3] Lowenstein PR, Castro MG "Evolutionary bass of a new gene- and immune-therapeutic approach for the treatment of malignant brain tumours: from mice to clinical trials for glioma patients" *Clin Immunol* 2018;189:43-51.

[4] Patil SA, Hosni-Ahmed A, Jones TS, Patil R, Pfeffer LM, Miller DD "Novel approaches to glioma drug design and drug screening" *Expert Opin Drug Discov* 2013;8(9):1135-51.

[5] Cordier D, Krolicki L, Morgenstern A, Merlo A "Targeted radiolabeled compounds in glioma therapy" *Semin Nucl Med* 2016;46(3):243-9.

[6] Miller JJ, Wen PY "Emerging targeted therapies for glioma" *Expert Opin Emerg Drugs* 2016;21(4):441-452.

[7] Oberheim Bush NA, Chang SM, Berger MS "Current and future strategies for treatment of glioma" *Neurosurg Rev* 2017;40(1):1-14.

[8] Peng Z, Liu C, Wu M "New insights into long noncoding RNAs and their roles in glioma" *Mol Cancer* 2018;17(1):61.

[9] Zhu C, Kros JM, Cheng C, Mustafa D "The contribution of timor-associated macrophages in glioma net-angiogenesis and implications for anti-angiogenic strategies" *Neuro Oncol* 2017;19(11):1435-1446.

[10] Tomiyama A, Ichimura K "Signal transduction pathways and resistance to targeted therapies in glioma" *Semin Cancer Biol* 2019;58:118-129.

[11] Li Shanshan, Ding Xia "TRPC channels and glioma" *Adv Exp Med Biol* 2017;965:157-165.

[12] GLASS Consortium "Glioma thought the looking GLASS: molecular evolution of diffuse gliomas and the glioma longitudinal analysis consortium" *Neuro Oncol* 2018;20(7):873-884.

[13] Sathornsumetee S, Rich JN "New treatment strategies for malignant gliomas" *Expert Rev Anticancer There* 2006;6(7):1087-104.

[14] van Tellingen O, Yetkin-Arik B, de Gooijer MC, Wesseling P, Wurdinger T, de Vries HE et al. "Overcoming the blood-brain tumour barrier for effective glioblastoma treatment" *Drug Resis Update* 2015;19:1-12.

[15] Patel M, Vogelbaum MA, Barnett GH, Jalali R, Ahluwalia MS "Molecular targeted therapy in recurrent glioblastoma: current challenges and future directions" *Expert Opin Investig Drugs* 2012;21(9):1247-66.

[16] Li B, Chang CM, Yuan M, McKenna WG, Shu HKG "Resistance to small molecule inhibitors of Epidermal growth factor receptor in malignant gliomas" *Cancer Res* 2003;63(21):7443-50.

Chapter 14

INFILTRATIVENESS ATTRIBUTES PROJECT SCHEMES OF ETIOLOGY AND PATHOGENESIS IN SEQUENTIAL MALIGNANT TRANSFORMATIONS IN GIVEN INDIVIDUAL GLIOMAS

ABSTRACT

Dynamics of tumor etiology and pathogenesis are prime consequences of multiple transformations derived directly from a realized evolutionary premise that suggests conversion of cell proliferative activity to systems of infiltrativeness of CNS tissues high grade gliomas. It is further to be considered that the infiltrativeness predeterminant is constitutional derivation of dysfunctional and homeostatic measures of the overall panorama of system biology of the evolutionary potentiality. Projection of novel biologic antigenicity outside the immune repertoire is a response by the organ and system immune systems. It is further to conclusive evidential derivation of a high grade glioma that transformational biology involves a pathogenesis that overshadows the implications of biologic system control; loss of glioma control is evolutional change of antigenicity of the individual tumor cells in integral neoplastic lesions.

Introduction

The diagnosis of a full range of primary brain tumors constitutes a challenge to therapeutic management of the patients in terms of the real potential for tumor response to immunotherapy. Inefficient delivery of immunostimulants across the blood-brain barrier is a main obstacle to overcome in induction of local immune responses in the brain [1]. The incremental progression of proliferation and spread of the tumor cells derives predetermined patterns of progression in constituting a non-operative response. A significant nonresponse within the system constitutional immune privilege of the central nervous system (CNS) is portrayed by patient outcome. Resting-state fMRI detects altered whole brain connectivity related to glioma biology [2].

Immune Non Response

The significant immune non-responsiveness of brain tumors in general is paramount consideration in terms that evolve further with increased progression of these lesions. It is further to such considerations that the immunity status of the CNS in specific terms conclusively predetermines aspects of biology of non-response within systems of appraised constitutional tumor pathogenesis. With the advances in single-cell RNA Sequencing, tumors can be dissected at the cell level, revealing multiple cell populations within tumors that drive evolution and treatment failure [3].

The constant crosstalk between the tumor microenvironment and the glioma cells determines the response to novel immunotherapies [4]. Radiomic profiles in high grade gliomas reveal distinct subtypes with prognostic import [5].

It is in terms of constitutional predetermination that the evolving biology of the individual neoplastic lesion induces significant deposition of tumor cells. Hierarchical restructuring of system biology are specific mechanics of the proliferation or spread phenomena. Integrin signaling is significant in glioma pathogenesis, formation of the tutor niche and brain tissue infiltration [6]. Constitutional etiologic derivation of the specific tumor lesion per se is significant attribute of the immune non- response. Myeloid-derived suppressor cells are a subset of immunosuppressive cells known to infiltrate the tutor microenvironment of glioblastoma; the CCL2-CCR2 axis is important for this process [7]. Surgical resection, radiotherapy or chemotherapy are inappropriate to specifically address the unique phenomena of tumor cell proliferation and spread within the CNS.

Attempts at Control

Derived assumptions in attempted control of spread of brain tumor spread is of phenomenal significance in terms that are constitutionally predetermined as an individual neoplasm in the biology of the whole integral lesion.

It is with a view to such predetermination that constitutional system biology is a predominant factor in causation of the lesion at the time of its causative origin within the CNS. Epidermal Growth Factor Receptor mutation is a novel prognostic factor related to immune infiltration in lower-grade glioma [8]. It is further to such considerations that the overwhelming potential causation of a given brain tumor is subservient to the evolving course of a lesion that primarily spreads rather than primarily proliferates. Tumor infiltrating lymphocytes and programmed death ligand 1 are targets for immune checkpoint inhibition; this is relevant for immune modulation in glioma patients [9].

Etiologic Measures

Tumor biology of non-response to currently employed therapeutic measures is hence a non-response as system mechanics that outline and further accentuate the spread and inclusive infiltration of CNS tissues. The distribution of timor-infiltrating T cells and PD-L1 expression has been reported in human gliomas; Interferon-gamma is an important cause of PD-L1 expression in the glioma microenvironment [10]. The immune-modulation that is inherent phenomenon systemically is a significant factor in the actual evolution of a neoplastic lesion that arises in terms primarily predetermined within the evolving etiologic mechanics of tumor progressiveness. Performance dynamics of evolving tumors are a significant mechanistic prerogative within the system biologic spread of the lesion within the CNS.

The significant recapitulation of lesion dysfunctionality is an aspect of integral evolution that specifically concentrates and focuses as predetermined infiltrativeness of high grade gliomas. In such terms, the further derivatives of operability as dictated by proliferation of spread are paramount attributes of the progressiveness of such infiltrativeness of the CNS tissues. The tumor microenvironment greatly modulates tumorogenesis, invasion and progression [11]. The ongoing derivation of such biologic predetermination is a predominant attribute that mechanistically evolves and reshapes immunotherapeutic potential for control of the subsequent pathogenetic course options of the individual brain tumor lesions. Combined anti-CXCR4 and anti-PD-1 immunotherapy provides survival benefit in glioblastoma through immune cell modulation of the tutor microenvironment [12].

Infiltrativeness

Predominance of infiltrativeness potentiality in progression of high grade gliomas is significant in terms of immunotherapeutic considerations in control of tumor system biology. The overall predeterminations are incremental dyshomeostatic mechanisms in the developmental history of a specific lesion that incorporates specific antigenic epitopes as endstage for infiltration of both grey and white matter of the CNS.

Glioblastoma has a low immunogenic response and an immunosuppressive microenvironment induced by the precise crosstalk between immune cells and cytokines [13].

The evolution of transformation of lesions that initially are etiologically active foci of transformation calls into operative dysfunction the performance dynamics of replacement biology as also determined along similar lines as embryologically predetermined. It is within successive performance dynamics of replacement that the high grade glioma induces the development of proliferative infiltrativeness of the neoplastic cell. Scattered data is available about the activity of immunosuppressive or immunostimulatory cell types in glioblastoma and these include tumor-associated macrophages, timor-infiltrating dendritic cells and regulatory T cells [14].

System and Organ Predetermination

System versus organ and cellular predetermination is a functional correlate of the cytokine systems in general, with a view towards the incorporation of lesion dysfunctions within homeostatic control systems of the CNS. The operative serial redefinitions of such potentialities of biologic dysfunction are hence the result of active homeostatic measures as borne out by the development of the initial evolution of the etiologically predetermined single focus of malignant transformation within the CNS.

Causation and Etiology

The causative factors in etiologic determination of infiltrativeness of the given neoplastic lesions are paramount evolutionary responses within the immune system itself rather than simply genetic factors in evolving pathologic predetermination of the integral high grade glioma.

Intern adhesion molecules and components of angiogenesis may potentially be useful as tumor progression markers and prognostic and diagnostic purposes [15]. In such terms, carcinogenesis is an attribute of constitutional import within considerations of derivation of the growth and spread of the tumor lesion. AMPA receptors enhance perivascular glioma invasion via beta1 integrin-dependent adhesion to the extracellular matrix [16]. Within system biology of dynamic cell turnover, the emergence of neoplasia is constitutionally an attribute that derives biologic earmarks of a lesion that primarily evolves as infiltration of the CNS tissues.

It is beyond considerations of derivation that the biology of tumors in general constitutes an active acquisition of new biologic attributes of evolving transformation. It is thus in terms of a whole sequence of transformations that the included carcinogenesis processes target evolutionary potentialities of simple homeostatic predetermination.

Conclusion

Substantial attributes of derivation of an individual high grade glioma as etiologically formulated are constitutional in terms of active operability issues of pathogenesis as further projected by a whole series of sequential homeostatic mechanisms within the CNS. It is further to such premises that the included integrity of a given tumor lesion predetermines constitutional attributes for carcinogenetic transformations. A given response as carcinogenic transformation implicates a whole system sequence of such transformations as projected within etiologic reformulations of such constitutional attributes. The further conformational derivatives are consequence restricted in terms that redefine each of the sequential transformations of tutor biology of the given neoplasm in terms that participate as infiltrativeness of the CNS tissues.

REFERENCES

[1] Yin P, Li H, Ke C, Cao G, Xin X, Hu J et al. "Intranasal delivery of immunotherapeutic nano formulations for treatment of glioma through in situ activation of immune response" *Int J Nanomedicine* 2020;15:1499-1515.

[2] Stoecklein VM, Stoecklein S, Galie F, Ren J, Schmutzer M, Unterrainer M et al. "Resting-state fMRI detects alterations in whole brain connectivity related to tumor biology in glioma patients" *Neuro Oncol* 2020;doi: 10.1093.

[3] Lopes MB, Vinga S "Tracking intratumor heterogeneity in glioblastoma via regulated classification of single-cell RNA-Seq data" *BMC Bioinformatics* 2020;21(1)doi:10.1186.

[4] Foray C, Barca C, Backhaus P, Schellhaas S, Winkler A, Viel T et al. "Multimodal molecular imaging of the tutor microenvironment" *Adv Exp Med Biol* 2020;1225:71-87.

[5] Lin P, Peng YT, Gao RZ, Wei Y, Li XJ, Huang SN et al. "Radiomic profiles in diffuse glioma reveal distinct subtypes with prognostic value" *J Cancer Res Clin Onco* 2020;146(5):1253-1262.

[6] Ellert-Miklaszewska A, Poleszak K, Pasierbinska M, Kaminska B "Integrin signaling in glioma pathogenesis: from biology to therapy" *Int J Mol Sci* 2020;21(3):888.

[7] Flores-Toro JA, Luo D, Gopinath A, Sarkisian MR, Campbell JJ, Charo I et al. "CCR2 inhibition reduces tumor myeloid cells and unmasks a checkpoint inhibitor effect to slow progression of resistant murine gliomas" *Proc Natl Acad Sci USA* 2020;117(2):1129-1138.

[8] Hao Z, Guo D "EGFR mutation: novel prognostic factor associated with immune infiltration in lower-grade glioma; an exploratory study" *BMC Cancer* 2019;19(1):1184.

[9] Berghoff AS, Kiesel B, Widhalm G, Wilheim D, Rajky O, Kurscheid S et al. "Correlation of immune phenotype with IDH mutation in diffuse glioma" *Neuro Oncol* 2017;19(11):1460-1468.

[10] Qian J, Wang C, Wang B, Yang J, Wang Y, Luo F et al. "The IFN-gamma/PD-L1 axis between T cells and tumor microenvironment:

hints for glioma anti-PD-1/PD-L1 therapy" *J Neuroinflammation* 2018;15(1):290.

[11] Chen J, Hou C, Wang P, Yang Y, Zhou D "Grade II/III glioma microenvironment mining and its prognostic merit" *World Neurosurg* 2019;132:doi:10.1016.

[12] Wu A, Maxwell R, Xia Y, Cardarelli P, Oyasu M, Belcaid Z et al. "Combination anti-CXCR4 and anti-PD-1 immunotherapy provides survival benefit in glioblastoma through immune cell modulation of tutor microenvironment" *J Neurooncol* 2019;143(2):241-249.

[13] Wang X, Guo G, Guan H, Yu Y, Lu J, Yu J "Challenges and potential of PD-1/PD-L1 checkpoint blockade immunotherapy for glioblastoma" *J Exp Clin Cancer Res* 2019;38(1):87.

[14] Antunes ARP, Scheyltjens I, Duerinck J, Neyns B, Movahedi K, Ginderachter JAV "Understanding the glioblastoma immune microenvironment as basis for the development of new immunotherapeutic strategies" *Elife* 2020;9doi:10.7554.

[15] Mizejewski GJ "Role of integrals in cancer: survey of expression patterns" *Proc Soc Exp Biol Med* 1999;222(2):124-38.

[16] Liao Y, Lu L, de Groot J "AMPA receptors promote perivascular glioma invasion via beta1 integrin-dependent adhesion to the extracellular matrix" *Neuro Oncol* 2009;11(3):260-73.

Chapter 15

PROGRESSIVELY PERSISTENT TUMOR CELL GROWTH AND RECURRENCE AND SPREAD AS INTERPLAY DYNAMICS BETWEEN INDIVIDUAL NEOPLASTIC CELLS

ABSTRACT

Interplay forces concern primarily increased growth of the individual tumor cells as these interact with other individual tumor cells. The recurrence phenomenon is simply a consequential derivative of the system biology systems of growth rather than of cell division within the encompassed consequence of immunosuppression. It is significant to view the hierarchical structuring of the neoplastic lesion as heterogeneous interplay between the individual tumor cells projected as recurrence and spread of the neoplasm.

INTRODUCTION

Substantial efforts in the understanding of solid tumors especially glioblastoma indicate that active immunosuppressive mechanisms reside both within the tumor cells and also in the tumor microenvironment. There is an interplay between senescence, autophagy and apoptosis in glioblastoma and this has direct impact in the understanding of tumor pathogenesis [1]. Alterations in tumor metabolism can contribute to a potent tolerogenic immune microenvironment with potential targeting of metabolic immune checkpoints as therapy for the tumor [2]. It is as a consequence of such pathway mechanisms that the overall derivation of all immunosuppressive processes kindles a series of ongoing pathways within the integral mechanics of tumor immunosuppression. In such terms, the effects of combinatorial and personalized dynamics involve necessity for recognition of complex interplay that also implicate the delivery of powerful but specific manipulative strategies in an attempt to control the effectiveness of incoming immune cells especially CD8+ T cells.

Summation Phenomena

The overall attributes of summation pathways are derivative properties of the system dimensions of integral antigen presentation. In such terms, the further increments of potentiality in immune activation are forward attribute as a first of tentative efforts for tumor control and eradication.

The distinctive dimensions of strict control of progression in cell growth and infiltration are requisite attributes that may bypass the encompassed eradication of the neoplasm. Extensive interplay occurs between Ephrin receptors, Rho GTPases and casein kinase 2 critical for understanding mechanisms of glioblastoma invasiveness [3]. It is significant to consider the free interplay of lesions within the tumor lesion as paramount recognition of complexity through simple dimensions of dynamic turnover of the neoplastic cells. IL-6 is released during microglia-glioblastoma crosstalk and induces barrier dysfunction due to the JAK/STAT3 pathway in endothelial cells and down regulation of intercellular junction proteins [4]. In such terms, the paradoxical growth of glioblastoma within the intracranial compartment is a significant attribute that may render the approaches to control for further growth and infiltration progression more effective. The dimensions for the development of mechanistic manipulation beside surgical resection are essential requirements in the development of effective therapy.

System Manipulation

The emergence of system pathway manipulation is hence a targeting strategy that should concern in particular the interplay and interaction manipulation of microenvironmental factors. In such terms, the microenvironment appears to potentially control biology of the glioblastoma cells.

It is further to such considerations that the incremental attributes of tumor cell growth and infiltration arise primarily within the immunosuppressive effects of the microenvironment. A complex interplay occurs between the glioblastoma genome and epigenome [5]. The system pathways of neoplastic biology are systems of increment in terms specific for the secondary attributes of individual and groups of tumor cells. The driven potentiality of tumor cells to progress is the specifically driven biology of systems of accumulation as biologic potentiality for carcinogenesis. There is interplay between neural stem cells and glioblastoma with a possible role of neurotrophic signaling. It is significant to realize the dimensions of immunosuppression as primary and derived attributes of such driven tumor growth and spread. Circular SMARCA5 RNA inhibits migration of glioblastoma cells by modulating a molecular axis involving splicing factors serine and arginine rich slicing factor 3 and 1 and of polypyrimidine tract binding protein 1 [6]. The further dimensions for realization of strict control without specific considerations of actual eradication of the neoplastic lesion include the transition of the microenvironment towards scope for further tumor growth. The further cooperative interplay may be considered to include the relative dynamics of integrally individual tumor cells within such a heterogeneous lesion as glioblastoma.

Performance Dynamics

Performance dynamics are a potential clue to pathogenesis of tumors in general and may include tumor cell replacement within clonal proliferation profiles of the individual glioblastoma lesion. In such terms, turnover dynamics are integral to specific growth attributes of the tumor, with the improviso that eradication of the lesion is a further potential target in neoplastic evolution. Immune checkpoint blockade has revolutionised cancer therapy but not in glioblastoma [7]. It is further to such concept that the further dimensions for tumor growth are themselves the derived sustained persistence of strict recurrence after subtotal surgical resection. Isocitrate dehydrogenase mutations influences global hypermethylation and patient prognosis and also degree of immune infiltration within individual tumors [8]. According to such a concept, the later evolution of a given glioblastoma are tentative attempts within the framework of system manipulation of immune responses to the growing tumor cells that divide in terms of biology of recurrence and tumor cell replacement. A complex interplay exits between tumor cell invasion and treatment resistance in glioblastoma and this impacts on new therapeutic approaches [9], Glioblastoma cancer stem cells appear to be neither resistant nor susceptible to chemotherapy per se [10]. Glioblastoma patients exhibit various levels of the elevated expression of DNA repair enzyme [10].

Tumor Growth Persistence

Considering the overall increment in progression of tumor cells is a particular property that sharply demarcates and further accentuates the dynamics of tumor growth and spread in terms of biologic recurrence. Glioblastoma cells are resistant to apoptotic stimuli and their death occurs through autophagy [11]. It is necessary to identify novel biomarkers associated with autophagy in glioblastoma [12]. The overall development of systems biology pathways are derived phenomena of the tumor microenvironment as exemplified by the emergence of infiltration with or without cell division. The system dynamics for further progression in tumor growth and spread simply multiply as terms of immunosuppression.

Autophagy is unregulated during stress conditions and in response to anti-cancer therapy; it regulates pro-growth signaling and metabolic processes of cancer cells in order to support tutor growth [13]. The question arises as to the existence of threshold doses for temozolomide that activate the death pathway and initiate apoptosis [14].

The possible attributes of immune surveillance are systems of recognition of specific tumor antigens in the first instance. The emergence for persistent neoplastic growth is hence the underlying framework for immunosuppression and is also a basis for recurrence of the tumor.

Such biologic drive in tumor progressiveness is an attribute that specifically reveals the interplay dimensions of tumor biology in terms of cooperative projection between individual tumor cells. In such terms, the microenvironment appears to provide the distributive potentialities for further growth and spread of the neoplasm. Recurrence of the lesion results within the dynamics of such interplay between individual tumor cells as derived phenomenon for further growth drive. Biology of systems for tumor recurrence is hence the attribute assignment for further growth with acceleration driven within dimensions for infiltration of the adjacent brain parenchyma.

CONCLUSION

The potentiality for specific control of tumor cell growth is the attribute designation of antitumor immune responses on the one hand and of a cooperative dimension for interplay between individual tumor cells. It is within the overall incremental growth of the lesion that infiltration further accentuates the derived system of recurrence of a subtotal resection.

Performance dimension is clearly a system determining pathways relative to potentiating attributes of tumor cell growth and spread. The incremental tumor progression is hence a realization of unresolved injury to cellular homeostatic mechanisms as further projected by genetic mutation in the manipulative evolution of primary and secondary systems of expressed immunosuppression and tumor cellular interplay.

REFERENCES

[1] Pawlowska E, Szczepanska J, Szatkowska M, Blasiak J "An interplay between senescence, apoptosis and autophagy in glioblastoma multiforme—role in pathogenesis and therapeutic perspective" *Int J Mol Sci* 2018;19(3):889.

[2] Kesarwani P, Kant S, Prabhu A, Chinnaiyan P "The interplay between metabolic remodelling and immune regulation in glioblastoma" *Neuro Oncol* 2017;19(10):1308-1315.

[3] de Gooijer MC, Navarro MG, Bernards R, Wurdinger T, van Tellingen O "An experimenter's guide to glioblastoma invasion pathways" *Trends Mol Med* 2018;24(9)763-780.

[4] Couto M, Coelho-Santos V, Santos L, Fontes-Ribeiro C, Silva AP, Gomes CMF "The interplay between glioblastoma and microglia cells leads to endothelial cell monolayer dysfunction via the interleukin-6-induced JAK2/STAT3 pathway" *J Cell Physiol* 2019;234(11):19750-19760.

[5] Sturm D, Bender S, Jones DTW, Lichter P, Grill J, Becher O et al. "Paediatric and adult glioblastoma: multiform (epi) genomic culprits emerge" *Nat Rev Cancer* 2014;14(2):92-107.

[6] Barbagallo D, Caponnetto A, Cirnigliaro M, Brex D, Barbagallo C, D'Angeli F et al. "CircSMARCA5 inhibits migration of glioblastoma multiforme cells by regulating a molecular axis involving splicing factors SRSF1/SRSF3/PTB" *Int J Mol Sci* 2018;19(2):480.

[7] Saha D, Martuza R, Rabkin SD "Oncolytic herpes simplex virus immunovirotherapy in combination with immune checkpoint blockade to treat glioblastoma" *Immunotherapy* 2018;10(9):779-786.

[8] Abedalthagafi M, Barakeh D, Foshay KM "Immunogenetics of glioblastoma: the future of personalised patient management" *NPJ Precis Oncol* 2018;2:27.

[9] Vollmann-Zwerenz A, Leidgens V, Feliciello G, Klein CA, Hau P "Tumor cell invasion in glioblastoma" *Int J Mol Sci* 2020;21(6):1932.

[10] Kohsaka S, Takahashi K, Wang L, Tanino M, Kimura T, Nishihara H "Inhibition of GSH synthesis potentiates temozolomide-induced bystander effect in glioblastoma" *Cancer Lett* 2013;331(1):68-75.

[11] Koukourakis MI, Mitrakas AG, Giatromanolaki A "Therapeutic interactions of autophagy with radiation and temozolomide in glioblastoma: evidence and issues to resolve" *Br J Cancer* 2016;114(5):485-96.

[12] Wang Y, Zhao W, Xiao Z, Gian G, Liu X, Zhuang M "A risk signature with four autophagy-related genes for predicting survival of glioblastoma multiforme" *J Cell Mol Med* 2020;24(7):3807-3821.

[13] Simpson JE, Gammon N "The impact of autophagy doing the development and survival of glioblastoma" *Open Biol* 2020;10(9):200184.

[14] He Y, Kaina B "Are there thresholds in glioblastoma cell death responses triggered by temozolomide?" *Int J Mol Sci* 2019;28(7):1562.

Chapter 16

Non-Response of the Immune System as Active Participant in Glioma Cell Genesis, Proliferation, and Spread in Normal Brain Tissues

Abstract

Promotional agent formulation is an actively acquired reformulation in gliomagenesis as defined in terms of a predominant phenomenon of the individual glioma cell infiltrating normal brain tissues. The emergence of injury to the tumor cell genome is hallmark phenomenon within a contrasting context that allows an active permissive microenvironment within which the lesion both proliferates and spreads. Derivative phenomena of non-response by immune systems as further propagated by suppression of schemes of non-acquisition contrast with dual pathways of actively employed systems in terms of the individual infiltrating neoplastic cell.

INTRODUCTION

The incremental progression of a glioma is a direct derivative dysfunctionality of the process of initiation of the lesion in terms of induced instigation of a transformational series of changes inherent to responding and non-responding parameters. Gliomagenesis in Neurofibromatosis 1 results in a heterogeneous spectrum of low- to high-grade neoplasms occurring throughout the entire lifespan of patients; in general, the profiling of NF1-glioma is defined by a distinct landscape that recapitulates a sub-group of sporadic tumors [1]. These arise as inherent attributes of the acquired dimensions of proliferative infiltrativeness of the individual tumor cell. As such, inclusive biologic traits of tumor cells dominant in an all-or-nothing phenomenon of progressiveness contrast within compound repetitive redefinition of pathways of non-resolution. The unique composition and functions of infiltrating and resident myeloid cells in glioblastoma establish a rationale to target infiltrating cells in this tumor-type [2]. In human glioblastoma, cadherin 4 can also actively contribute in the modulating regulation of cell invasiveness and malignancy [3]. Hence, terms of reference inherently arising particularly within contextual phenomena of inclusiveness of the infiltration events allow for emergence of non-antigenicity of the parent lesion at its inception.

NONRESPONSE

The parameters of non-response on the part of immune competent cells and of immune humoral factors are testimonial evidence towards a phenomenon of acquisition of novel capabilities of biologic import. In addition to cell autonomous signaling functions, the neurotrophins and their respective receptors contribute to drive the cellular and molecular composition of the glioma microenvironment, thus promoting tumorigenesis [4]. It is in the realization of infiltration of normal brain tissues that dynamics of emergence of gliomagenesis perpetuate within shifting dependency requirements in terms especially of immune suppression. Intratumor heterogeneity in glioblastoma is a conserved predictable consequence to its complex microenvironment, and evolutionary cues drive gliomagenesis as conserved molecular events [5]. In such terms, ongoing biologic formulas of perpetuation of growth and expansion of the primary tumor mass are relevant to a process of progressive tumor spread. Neuropathology assessment of gliomas rely increasingly on ancillary testing of molecular alterations for proper patient management [6]. It is beyond such infiltrative phenomena that tumor grade is derived index of progression of infiltration beyond the parent process of initial gliomagenesis. NF-kappaB activating protein alters tumor immune microenvironment and promotes glioma growth via Notch1 signaling [7].

PATHOGENIC PATHWAYS

Binary and parallel pathogenetic pathways of non-resolution of the progressive infiltrativeness of individual tumor cells stand in paradoxical contrast with a proliferativeness of parent neoplastic cells that fail to elicit an immune response directed against the expanding glioma. Blocking the potential sources of glioma stem cells and improving the local tumor -inducing and -promoting microenvironment appears indicated beyond simple eradication of the existing glioma stem cells [8]. In such context, the central nervous system both participates and also suppresses the immune response to the neoantigenicity of both the tumor mass cells and also the infiltrating individual tumor cells. In such terms, ongoing development of the lesion as a primary mechanism of spreading infiltration is paramount derivative of the surrounding normal CNS tissues that both provoke and sustain the further gliomagenesis. Elucidating epigenetic control is essential to understanding glioblastoma biology beyond signature mutational profiles [9].

Perforce increments as progression of the tumor are performance hallmarks of a system of active acquisition of biologic redefinitions in the contextual relative emergence of a glioma-genetic phenomenon. It is within the system biology of acquired insult to the genetic apparatus of emerging glioma cells, that there is instituted pathways of non- resolution of the immune response to the infiltrating tumor cells.

The emergence as dictated neoantigenicity is a unique parameter that suppresses and further evolves in terms of such failed immune surveillance of the peripheral and central antigen-presenting cells to the tumor. Isocitrate dehydrogenase gene mutation occurs in the early stages of gliomagenesis and contributes to suppression of the immune response [10]. Incremental emergence of gliomagenesis is inherent product formulation as best exemplified by dynamics of the infiltrative individual glioma cell. Immunologic sub-typing of glioblastoma is necessarily indicated to identify patients who may benefit from immune checkpoint therapy, including TNFSF14 as a significant adverse prognostic factor [11].

Normal Infiltrated Tissues

Normal brain tissues are relevant formulas as significant participants within redefinitions of systems of promoted induction phenomena. Suppression biology is indeed the central player in the inclusive definition of the individual tumor cell that infiltrates and progresses also as incremental size of the parent neoplastic lesion. The better realization of genetic injury to tumor cells is best achieved within the system conformation of non-immunogenicity of such defined tumorigenesis. The parameters of expansion contrast with a biology that is significant as inceptive formula of derived acquisition for further progression in growth and spread of the individual tumor cell.

Incremental Suppression

Formulations of increased suppression of the immune response to tumor neoantigenicity allow for a progression inherently manifesting as pathways of non-resolution of both the gliomagenesis and of the non-immunogenicity of acquired dimensions. PD-L1 is unregulated in glioblastoma and acts synergistically with other checkpoint members; it is associated with T-cell activation and macrophage-related immune responses and produces worse patient survival [12]. Realization of injury to systems is referable as infiltrativeness beyond pathways of cumulative formulas. Methylation signatures have been identified that classify different subtypes of diffuse glioma and the signatures may complement the WHO classification scheme of diffuse glioma [13]. Dynamics of normal brain tissue cells are receptive and also agonist participants within the reframed derivative formulas of spread in the form of the individual infiltrating glioma cells. Multiplicity of suppressive pathways in immune nonresponse allows the emergence of permissive system biology as defined by mechanistic considerations.

Neoantigenicity

The strictly operative process of essential biologic acquisition of neoantigenicity of the tumor cells is a system acquisition of the suppressive immune status as defined by infiltration of normal brain tissue.

In such terms, ongoing participation of the essentially dividing tumor cell is paramount receptive phenomenon within both proliferation and infiltrativeness, as exhibited by high-grade gliomas and as further exhibited by conclusive dimensions of non-resolution in terms of the suppression of the immune response. Peripheral immune status is relevant to considerations of an infiltrativeness that promotes interactivity with the normal brain tissues. Telomerase reverse transcriptase promoter mutation is dependent on tumor grade and the iso-citrate dehydrogenase mutational status in prognosis [14].

Contextual Reformulations

Contextual reformulations of interactivity include the inherent nature of a glioma that is system pathway for more incremental growth and spread of the individual tumor cell. Since transcriptional class is only partially explained by underlying genomic alterations, the tumor microenvironment may also have an impact [15]. The participation of genetic lesions is subservient formula that includes cumulative creation of further lesions as projected by high-grade gliomas. The strict definition of such injuries arise within the proficient participation of non-response as dictated paradoxically by actively proliferating and spreading neoplastic cells. It is with such formula of emergence in gliomagenesis that the significant spread of the tumor cells is directly defining term in the process of inception of further tumor cell genesis.

Microenvironment and genetics can both drive mesenchymal transcriptional signature in glioblastoma [16].

The significant biology of immune non-responsiveness is hence an inducive definition in interactions with the normal brain tissues and as redefined repeatedly in terms of infiltrated brain tissues. Neurofibromin1 deficient glioblastoma frequently shows a mesenchymal gene expression signature indicating a possible relationship between NF1 status and the tumor microenvironment; production of secreted cytokines/chemokines occurs in NF1 -deficient glioma [17].

Conclusion

Non-immunogenicity is a strictly parent and inherent attribute within the agonist systems of acquisition of glioma biology, as further projected by the infiltrating individual glioma cell. Pathogenic mutations in neurofibromin identifies a leucine-rich domain modulating glioma cell invasiveness [18]. In such terms promotion of suppressive biology is system definition as indicated by inclusive formulas of proliferation and spread of the neoplastic cells. It is further to be realized that fundamental acquisition of neoantigenicity participates as system formula in the progressive gliomagenesis of the expanding primary tumor lesion. The contrasting active acquisition of aggressive biologic traits of a high-grade glioma contrasts with redefined suppressive phenomena of the immune response.

Such suppressive immunogenicity is parent term in contributing to the active acquisition of a tumor biology beyond system-redefined attributes. The realization of gliomagenesis arises in terms derived from normal tissue infiltration, as further evidence of a novel microenvironmental permissiveness further defined by the non-response of the immune response.

REFERENCES

[1] D'Angelo F, Ceccarelli M, Tala, Garofano L, Zhang J, Frattini V et al. "The molecular landscape of glioma in patients with Neurofibromatosis 1" *Nat Med* 2019;25(1):176-187.

[2] Chen Z, Feng X, Herting CJ, Garcia VA, Nie K, Pong WW et al. "Cellular and molecular identity of tumor-associated macrophages in glioblastoma" *Cancer Res* 2017;77(9):2266-2278.

[3] Ceresa D, Alessandrini F, Bosio L, Marubbi D, Reverberi D, Malatesta P et al. "Cdh4 down-regulation impairs in vivo infiltration and malignancy in patients derived glioblastoma cells" *Int J Mol Sci* 2019;20(16):4028.

[4] Alshehri MM, Robbins SM, Senger DL "The role of neurotrophic singling gliomagenesis: a focus on the p75 neurotrophic receptor (p75NTR/CD271)." *Vitam Horm* 2017;104:356-404.

[5] Prabhu A, Kesarwani P, Kant S, Graham SF, Chinnaiyan P "Histologically defined intratumoral sequencing uncovers evolutionary cues into conserved molecular events driving gliomagenesis" *Neuro Oncol* 2017;19(12):1599-1606.

[6] Appin CL, Brat DJ "Molecular pathways in gliomagenesis and their relevance to neuropathologic diagnosis" *Adv Anat Pathol* 2015;22(1):50-8.

[7] Gu G, Gao T, Zhang L, Chen X, Pang Q, Wang Y et al. "NKAP alters tumor immune microenvironment and promotes glioma growth via Notch1 signaling" *J Exp Clin Cancer Res* 2019;38(1):291.

[8] Dong J, Huang Q "Targeting glioma stem cells: enough to terminate gliomagenesis?" *Chin Med J* (Engl) 2011;124(17):2756-63.

[9] Fomchenko EI, Erson-Omay EZ, Zhao A, Bindra RS, Huttner A, Fulbright RK et al. "DNMT3A co-mutation in an IDH1-mutant glioblastoma" *Cold Spring Harb Mol Case Stud* 2019;5(4):a994119.

[10] Gao M, Lin Y, Liu X, Li Y, Zhang C, Wang Z et al. "ISG20 promotes local tumor immunity and contributes to poor survival in human glioma" *Oncoimmunology* 2018;8(2):e1534038.

[11] Long S, Li M, Liu J, Yang Y, Li G "Identification of immunologic subtype and prognosis of GBM based on TNFSF14 and immune checkpoint gene expression profiling" *Aging* (Albany NY) 2020;12(8):7112-7128.

[12] Wang Z, Zhang C, Liu X, Wang Z, Sun L, Li G et al. "Molecular and clinical characterisation of PD-L1 expression at transcriptional level via 976 samples of brain glioma" *Oncoimmunology* 2016;16;5(11):e1195310.

[13] Paul Y, Mondal B, Patil V, Somasundaram K "DNA methylation signatures for 2016 WHO classification subtypes of diffuse gliomas" *Clin Epigenetics* 2017;9:32.

[14] Vuong HG, Alibi AMA, Duong UNP, Ngo HTT, Pham TQ, Chan AK-Y et al. "TERT promoter mutation and ints interaction with IDH mutations in glioma: combined TERT promoter and IDH mutations stratifies lower-grade glioma into distinct survival subgroups-A

Meta-analysis of aggregate data" *Crit Rev Oncol Hematol* 2017;120:1-9.

[15] Cooper LAD, Gutman DA, Chisolm C, Appin C, Kong J, Rong Y et al. "The tumor microenvironment strongly impacts master transcriptional regulators and gene expression class of glioblastoma" *Am J Pathol* 2012;180(5):2108-19.

[16] Orr BA, Eberhart CG "Nature versus nurture in glioblastoma: microenvironment and genetics can both drive mesenchymal transcriptional signature" *Am J Pathol* 2012;180(5):1768-71.

[17] Wood MD, Mukherjee J, Pieper RO "Neurofibromin knockdown in glioma cell lines is associated with changes in cytokine and chemokine secretion in vitro" *Sci Rep* 2018;8(1):5805.

[18] Fadhlullah SFB, Halim NBA, Yeo JYT, Ho RLY, Um P, Ang BT et al. "Pathogenic mutations in neurofibromin identifies a leucine-rich domain regulating glioma cell invasiveness" *Oncogene* 2019;38(27):5367-5380.

Chapter 17

PATHWAYS OF NON-RESOLUTION IN TARGETING TUMOR CELLS BY THE IMMUNE RESPONSE

ABSTRACT

Lymphocyte turnover as a selective and specific mechanistic pathway in the amplification of the immune response is based on a concept of realized antigenicity within systems for further stimulation of immunity towards the tumor cells. It is in such terms that targeting events are dominant pathways as further confirmed by systems of facilitated antigenicity and as further dimensionalized within the character participation of costimulatory molecules, on the one hand, and the possible multiplicity of tumor related antigenicity.

INTRODUCTION

Processing and presentation of antigen are a fundamental series of mechanisms that constitute the integral dimensions of realization of the activation of T cells within the added context of alternative endogenous or exogenous pathways of involvement by antigen presenting cells.

Members of the major facilitator superfamily of transport proteins are critical for the movement of a wide range of substrates across biomembranes [1]. The up regulation of glucose transporters has been described in several cancer types as a result of perturbation of gene expression or protein relocalization or stabilisation [2]. In such terms, the overall rendering of T cells within the lymph node selective zones for T cells and follicular germinal centers is product mechanisms within the added MHC/peptide restriction and costimulatory molecular apparatuses. There is emerging evidence that tumor-derived exosomes can construct a fertile environment to support tumor proliferation, angiogenesis, invasion and premetastatic niche preparation [3].

The significance of such derivative phenomena includes the development of the precise processing/activation within professional APC (antigen presenting cells) that promote significant anticipation of lymphocyte activation.

Promotional dynamics of activation of APC correlate with activation of lymphocyte subsets, including in particular CD8+ and CD4+ T lymphocytes. In such manner the problematic dimension for cooperative involvement of cytokines, on the one hand, and of specific receptor targeting include a critical realization within systems of amplification of target cell specificity, especially as applicable for T lymphocytes. Although host cells die at low extracellular pH, cancer cells resist, as they are well equipped with transporters and enzymes to regulate intracellular pH homeostasis [4]. The success of anti-tumor immune responses depends on the infiltration of solid tumors by effector T cells, a process guided by chemokines [5]. With regard to definitive cooperation with a series of cytokine contexts allowing for the lymphocyte activation and targeting of the tumor cells, the product series of mechanisms are permissive within the system profiles of ongoing turnover of the T lymphocytes.

Contextual Antigen Restriction

The realization of ongoing contextual restriction by MHC in cells is antigen dependent within the further system profiles of ongoing cellular turnover. Rational strategies for combination immunotherapy expand and promote the trafficking of tumor-specific T cells [6].

Therapeutic monoclonal antibodies targeting immune checkpoints have changed the treatment landscape of many tumors; a major factor involved in initial resistance to immune checkpoint inhibitors is the lack or paucity of tumor cell infiltration [7].

The transport of antigen within the cytosol of APC is dependent systems of molecular binding that in turn involve the participation of moderate to strong affinities as evidenced by involvement of the proteasome degrading systems and the dimensions of the functional endoplasmic reticulum.

System Co-Stimulation

In similar terms, direct or indirect presentation to T lymphocytes allows for the implication of system profiles as reflected by CD8+ and CD4+ T lymphocyte subsets. It is further to such realization that the mechanistic promotion of antigen targeting to the lymphocyte is integral to the functional cooperation of a range of cytokine and costimulatory molecules within systems of preference as reflected by protocol profiles of selective promotion of the central lymphocyte activation/targeting mechanisms.

Cooperative progression of the immune response requires the maintenance of targeting as projected by the end result of dimensional states of activation of the lymphocytes in terms of specificity and cellular subset selectivity and of induced response to tumor cells. Tumor cells constitute poor APC but implicate other effector mechanisms, including B lymphocytes and macrophages.

Natural killer cells, on the other hand, implicate the innate and nonspecific immune system and are involved in contexts of nonrestricted antigenicity with regard to the major histocompatibility complex (MHC).

Antigen Processing

Overall, dimensions of antigen processing are hence a setting stage that primarily selects amplification as indicated by MHC restricted antigen presentation. The involvement of disparate antigens indicates a whole heterogeneous series of promotional events towards the activation of various subsets of T lymphocytes. Chimeric antigen receptor autologous T cells encode an antigen-specific single-chain variable fragment and various costimulatory molecules; these modified T cells traffic to and recognise cancer cells in an HLA-independent manner [8]. A realization for the emergence of an immune response is clearly the activation of intracellular transport as denoted by the further development of partially processed antigen. Indeed, the significant emergence of lymphocyte activation foreshadows the performance of targeting as a dominant series of effector mechanisms in the evolution of the tumor cell directed immune response.

Immunologic Memory

Memory for immunologic specificity includes the performance attributes of targeting of the MHC restricted antigenicity as result effector pathways within the systems of realization of the immune response.

A hierarchical series of promotional facilitation and the rapid institution of the immune response are dictated within systems of performance of such memory dynamics. The overall implications of memory dynamics are further promotional realization as conveyed by systems of preference of both selectivity and specificity. Lack of CD103+ dendritic cells within the tumor microenvironment dominantly resists the defector phase of an anti-tumor T cell response, contributing to immune escape [9]. Inefficient infiltration of activated cytotoxic T lymphocytes into established tumors is increasingly being recognised as one of the major hurdles limiting efficacy [10]. It is further to the implications of molecular restriction as conveyed by the MHC complex bound to partially degraded peptides that there evolves lymphocyte turnover and transport to lymph nodes and spleen.

MOLECULAR TARGETING

Conclusive integrals within the various effector mechanisms allow for the emergence of cooperative dimensions as conveyed by systems of molecular physical configuration. This particularly applies to the evolutionary dynamics of the immune response. T cell migration across vascular endothelium is essential for T cell responses, as through the expression of specific tissue-homing receptors [11]. The memory instants for cooperative involvement implicate an ongoing maintenance as formulated for the regression of the tumor.

T cells genetically engineered to express chimeric antigen receptors have proven and impressive therapeutic activity in B cell leukaemia or lymphoma subtypes with also promising efficacy in multiple myeloma. Key challenges include severe toxicities, restricted trafficking to, infiltration into and activation within tumors, suboptimal persistence in vivo, antigen escape and heterogeneity [12].

The multiplicity of effector pathways and the diversity in some cases of endogenous and exogenous processing within APC are a reflected phenomenon that promotes the tumor targeting. Suppression of the anti-tumor immune response that is invariably ongoing is paramount consideration in the failure of the immune response to target the tumor cells. Soluble tumor antigens in particular are permissive within contexts of the immune response that specifically fails to induce tumor regression.

Conclusion

The ongoing realization at generating an amplifying series of targeting events in terms of anti-tumor regression is dependent on the emergence of significant participation of compound molecular constitution as further projected in terms of targeting events. The identity promotion of facilitated immune response allows for the participation of activated lymphocytes and also of the innate immune system. In terms of such ongoing attempts, maintenance of such immune response would also include self antigens as collaborative dimensions for recognition of tumor antigenicity per se.

It is further to such considerations that overall promotion of facilitated amplification of tumor antigenicity is a central concern as realized within pathways of constitutive molecular antigen targeting and of activation of lymphocytes that are persistently undergoing cellular turnover.

Promotional protocols of antigen amplification lies at the center of a series of intersecting effector pathways as further compounded by facilitated memory induced participation of the immune response and of the realization of both direct and indirect pathways of molecular degradation of the antigens arising and released or secreted by the tumor.

References

[1] Quistgaard EM, Low C, Guettou F, Nordlund P "Understanding transport by the major facilitator superfamily (MFS): structures pave the way" *Nat Rev Mol Cell Biol* 2016;17(2):123-32.

[2] Ancey PB, Contat C, Meylan E "Glucose transporters in cancer—from tumor cells to the tumor microenvironment" *FEB J* 2018;285(16):2926-2943.

[3] Wang Z, Chen JQ, Liu JL, Tian L "Exosomes in tumor microenvironment: novel transporters and biomarkers" *J Transl Med* 2016;14(1):297.

[4] Payen VL, Hau MY, Radecke KS, Wyart E, Vazeille T, Boutin C et al. "Monocarboxylate transporter MCT1 promotes tumor metastasis independently of its activity as a lactate transporter" *Cancer Res* 2017;77(20): 5591-5601.

[5] Barreira da Silva R, Laird ME, Yatim N, Fiette L, Ingersoll MA, Albert ML "Dipeptidylpeptidase 4 inhibition enhances lymphocyte trafficking, improving both naturally occurring tutor immunity and immunotherapy" *Nat Immunol* 2015;16(8):850-8.

[6] Camino-Mathews A, Foote JB, Emens LA "Immune targeting in breast cancer" *Oncology* (Williston Park) 2015;29(5):375-85.

[7] Bonaventura P, Shekarian T, Alcazar V, Valladeau-Guilemond J, Valsesia-Wittmann S, Amigorena S et al. "Cold tutors: a therapeutic challenge for immunotherapy" *Front Immune* 2019;10:168.

[8] Yoku O, Li X, Brentjens RJ "Adoptive T-cell therapy for solid tumors" *Am Soc Clin Oncol Educ Book* 2017;37:193-204.

[9] Stranger S, Dai D, Horton B, Gajewski TF "Tumor-residing Batf3 dendritic cells are required for effector T cell trafficking and adoptive T cell therapy" *Cancer Cell* 2017;31(5):711-723.

[10] Sharma RK, Chheda ZS, Jala VR, Haribabu B "Regulation of cytotoxic T-lymphocyte trafficking to tumors by chemoattractants: implications for immunotherapy" *Expert Rev Vaccines* 2015;14(4):537-49.

[11] Chimen M, Apta BH, Mcgettrick HM "Introduction: T cell trafficking in inflammation and immunity" *Methods Mol Biol* 2017;1591:73-84.

[12] Rafiq S, Hackett CS, Brentjens RJ "Engineering strategies to overcome the current roadblocks in CAR T cell therapy" *Nat Rev Clin Oncol* 2020;17(3):147-167.

Chapter 18

TUMOR CELL ANTIGENICITY AS PERFORMANCE HIERARCHY OF EQUILIBRATING INTERACTIVITY OF SYSTEMS OF RECEPTIVITY AND ACTIVATION OF LYMPHOCYTE SUBSETS

ABSTRACT

A multifold dimensionality within equilibrating performance of the immune response belies the development of hierarchical dimensions as conveyed by development of evolutionary dynamics of such immune response. The realization of significance in activation of both helper and cytotoxic T lymphocytes reflects the complexity of immunogenicity as a web-wide dimension in the further projection of injury to systems of tumor proliferation and infiltration of brain tissue. It is perhaps within systems of enhanced participation of tumor cell release of antigens that there exists the equilibration performance for further modification of the immune response towards tumor dynamics and cell constitutive series of antigen identities.

INTRODUCTION

The scope of introduction and maturation of dendritic cells constitutes the harnessing of a multi-potent derivative of circulating and bone marrow progenitors as termed professional antigen-presenting cells. Studies suggest improved overall survival and of progression free survival with dendritic cell therapy [1]. Immunotherapy shows great promise in patients with high-grade glioma [2, 3]. In the realization of injury to tumor cells in general and of intracranial brain tumors in particular, it is significant to consider dendritic cells within a body-wide web of receptor and effector cells borne out by systems of recognition of antigen presentation [4]. In such terms the incremental derivation of antigen presence is inherently linked to activation of the naïve lymphocytes as significantly projected by lymphoid tissue and thymus. Recent trials have shown that dendritic cells promote an anti-tumor immune response and sensitize glioma cells to chemotherapy [5]. The development of derivation dynamics is further enhanced as portrayed by dynamics of expansion of the dendritic cells that can be accomplished ex vivo.

ANTIGEN DERIVATION

Pronounced derivation of antigen processing and presentation is central to a whole series of tumor cell extract recognition as evidenced by systems for further activation and proliferation of both CD4+ T cells and of cytotoxic CD8+ cells. It may be necessary to evaluate molecular genetic abnormalities in individual patient tumors formulate novel immunotherapeutic strategies [6]. In such terms, the performance attributes of antigen presentation provoke the evolutionary development of immune activation within systems of proliferation and spread of brain tumor cells. Peptide-based immunotherapy could be a new treatment modality in patients with glioma [7]. It is further to such considerations that the escape phenomenon of antigens that are not recognized by the immune systems evolves in terms of acquisition and repeated degradation of major histocompatibility complex molecules as portrayed within systems of enhanced recognition/sensitization of immune effector cells. Dendritic cells are potent initiators of adaptive immune responses and hence central players in immunotherapy [8].

WEAK ANTIGENICITY

The problematic weakness of antigenicity of tumor suppressor cells is paramount consideration of the realization of tumor antigen presentation to immune effector cells. Considering the heterogeneity of malignant gliomas and an immune-refractory tumor cell population, rational multiple modalities that target different characteristics of the neoplasm may prove the most effective therapeutic strategy [9]. In such terms, the overall dynamics of equilibrating processes of exchange and of cross presentation constitute evidential support to the endogenous versus exogenous presentation processes as directed to CD4+ T lymphocytes in particular. Insight into the complex dynamics of immune-tumor interactions promises to delineate mechanisms of immune synergy with other treatment modalities [10]. An equilibrating scenario of induced lymphocyte effector activation is predominant in the realization of a whole series of processing events that include in particular a series of co-stimulatory molecules on the tumor cell surface.

Composite dimensions as evidential processing of antigens is especially effective with regard to dendritic cells as further pronounced within systems of performance of activation phenomena specifically involving T lymphocytes. A number of immunobiologic features of the brain and of gliomas may critically affect the regulation of effective treatment, including the presence of the blood brain barrier and the lack of organised secondary lymphatic tissues, low expression of histocompatibility antigens and the presence of immunosuppressants produced by the glioma cells [11]. In terms of involvement of injury, the realization of bacteria and other extrinsic sources of foreign antigens constitutes a strict characterization of the dynamics of expression of tumor associated antigens per se. It is further to the embodied dimensions of lymphocyte activation that these constitute the development of effector roles for the immune system as integral whole series of web-based interactivities. Cross-talk occurs between T cells and hematopoietic stem cells during adoptive cellular therapy for high grade gliomas [12].

Equilibrating Performance

The equilibrating performance derivatives of antigen presentation by dendritic cells constitute the hierarchical system profile of the immune system as integral presentation dependence as borne out by the consequent evolutionary traits of effector immune system participation. Evidence supports a significant interplay between gliomagenesis and the immune system; CD8+ T-cell infiltrates are related to prolonged survival [13]. In such terms, constitutive response of the immunogenicity of tumor cells is a conditioned reappraisal phenomenon that performs multi functional activation within body wide web participation. The significance roles for a complex of pathogenetic pathways are well illustrated by the evolutionary role of antigen presentation that is primarily activating. It is performance dynamics of immunogenicity as a single step in antigen-presentation phenomena that constitute the realization of pathways of adverse dimensions; this is illustrated by the possible emergence of autoimmune demyelination as a toxic byproduct in the constitution of the immunogenicity as offered by tumor cell beds and in particular by infiltrating tumor cells.

Systems of Activation

Equilibrating and recognition indices of activation of the immune system are a performance dynamics that incorporates dendritic cells as a specific web-based activity. Adjuvant immunotherapy utilising whole-cell sate dendritic cell vaccine may extent short-term survival [14]. It is paramount to consider weak antigenicity of tumor cells in terms of constitutional equilibration as presented by cell surface receptivity in the first instance. In such terms, ongoing derivation of lymphocyte activation perform a realization of stimulated and co-stimulated forces as portrayed by a whole series of cytokine production and secretion of effector lymphocytes.

CONCLUSION

The derivational dynamics of lymphocyte activation are performance attributes of antigen presentation by dendritic cells in particular and as evidenced by systems of provoking profile within body-wide web activity.

The field of immunotherapy is advancing in terms of the active specific immunotherapy utilising autologous dendritic cells as vehicle for immunisation [15].

The antigenicity derivative formulas are depicted by the emergence of constitutional immunity that first recognizes foreign antigens and then processes such antigens in terms of tumor cell immunogenicity. It is further to considerations of such performance that the immune system is primarily antigen-presenting within a strict hierarchy of constitutional equilibration of endogenous and exogenous derived presentation of such antigens. Dendritic cells are essential for priming but ineffective for boosting antitumor immune response in a murine model of glioma [16].

Significant property for change in activation status is further projected as immune derivation of partly processed or fragmented antigens within systems receptive for further stimulation of anti-glioma injury as constituted by infiltrating tumor cells within the central nervous system. The realization of injury is significant within such hierarchical systems of interactivity as evidenced by performance dynamics of the immune response.

REFERENCES

[1] Vatu BI, Artene SA, Staicu AG, Turcu-Stiolica A, Folcuti C, Dragoi A et al. "Assessment of efficacy of dendritic cell therapy and viral therapy in high grade glioma clinical trials. A meta-analytic review" *J Immunoassay immunochem* 2019;40(1):70-80.

[2] Artene SA, Turcu-Stiolica A, Ciurea ME, Folcuti C, Tataranu LG, Alexandru O et al. "Comparative effect of immunotherapy and standard therapy in patients with high grade glioma: a meta-analysis of published clinical trials" *Sci Rep* 2018;8(1):11800.

[3] Cao JX, Zhang XY, Liu JL, Li D, Li JL, Liu YS et al. "Clinical efficacy of tumor antigen-pulsed DC treatment for high-grade glioma: evidence from a meta-analysis" *PLoS One* 2014;9(9):e107173.

[4] Wang X, Zhao HY, Zhang FC, Sun Y, Xiong ZY, Jiang XB "Dendrtic cell-based vaccine for the treatment of malignant glioma: a systematic review" *Cancer Invest* 2014;32(9):451-7.

[5] Luptrawan A, Liu G, Yu JS "Dentritic cell immunotherapy for malignant gliomas" *Rev Recent Clin Trials;* 3(1):10-21.

[6] Yamanaka R "Dendritic-cell- and peptide-based vaccination strategies for glioma" *Neurosurg Rev* 2009;32(3):265-73.

[7] Yamanaka R, Itoh K "Peptide-based immunotherapeutic approaches to glioma: a review" *Expert Opin Biol Ter* 2007;7(5):645-9.

[8] Filley A. Dey M "Dendritic cell based vaccination strategy: an evolving paradigm" *J Neurooncol* 2017;133(2):223-235.

[9] Akasaki Y, Black KL, Yu JS "T cell immunity in patients with malignant glioma: recent progress in dendritic cell-based immunotherapeutic approaches" *Front Biosci* 2005;10:2908-21.

[10] Wheeler CJ, Black KL "Dendritic cell vaccines and immunity in glioma patients" *Front Biosci* 2005;10:2861-81.

[11] Pollack IF, Okada H, Chambers WH "Exploitation of immune mechanisms in the treatment of central nervous system cancer" *Semin Podiatry Neural* 2000;7(2):131-43.

[12] Wildes TJ, Grippin A, Dyson KA, Wummer BM, Damiani DJ, Abraham RS et al. "Cross-talk between T cells and hematopoietic stem cells during adoptive cellular therapy for malignant glioma" *Clin Cancer Res* 2018;24(16):3955-3966.

[13] Yang I, Tihan T, Han SJ, Wrensch MR, Wiencke J, Sughrue ME et al. "CD8+ T-cell infiltrate in newly diagnosed glioblastoma is associated with long-term survival" *J Clin Neurosci* 2010;17(11):1381-5.

[14] Cho DY, Yang WK, Lee HC, Hsu DM, Lin HL, Lin SZ et al. "Adjuvant immunotherapy with whole-cell lysate dendritic cells vaccine for glioblastoma multiform: a phase II clinical trial" *World Neurosurg* 2012;77(5-6):736-44.

[15] Van Good S, Maes W, Ardon H, Verschuere T, V Cauter S, de Vkeeschouwer S "Dendritic cell therapy of high-grade gliomas" *Brain Pathol* 2009;19(4):694-712.

[16] Jouanneau E, Poujol D, Le Mercier I, Blay JY, Belin MF, Puisieux I "Dendritic cells are essential for priming but inefficient for boosting antitumor immune response in an orthotropic murine glioma model" *Cancer Immunol immunother* 2006;55(3):254-67.

Chapter 19

Systems of Primary Regional Reformation in Tumor Origin and Mechanics: Regional versus Field Operability

Abstract

Substantiality of the inclusion performance dynamics of proliferation of a primarily strict regional field involvement in the inception of a tumor such as a glioma are paramount inclusions as derivative dimensions for further spread and infiltration. In such terms, such reformation is contrasting indices to a simple single cell of origin concept for tumors in general. It is within mechanistic formulas of such origin and spread of a glioma that there emerges the incongruity of an infiltrative phenomenon that further comprises systems of vascularization and further spread of the neoplasm. Strict regional basis of tumorigenesis contrasts with a simple field operability and invokes vascularization as integral to gliomagenesis.

Introduction

Sensitization of highly proliferating glioma or tumor cells is a fundamental aim in the delivery of a series of radiotherapeutic modalities in a manner that complements surgical debulking. The impact of targeted therapies in glioma is clearly modest [1]. Investigations exploring the precise molecular mechanisms and reliable therapeutic targets for gliomas have drawn intense attention [2]. It is significant to consider the overall dimensions of incumbent tumor growth within a sphere of therapeutic efforts to control the local tumor dynamics as these latter specifically impact the dimensions of diffuse spread of the neoplastic cells. The involvement of altered metabolic pathways such as glycolysis, oxidative phosphorylation and glutaminolysis suggest new possibilities for treatment; the different aspects of metabolic reprogramming in gliomas relate to glioma cell biology and the wider tumor microenvironment [3]. The manner of involvement of such diffuse spread are themselves instigators in the persistent local growth of the primary tumor mass in a manner that translates as a marked tendency for recurrence of the neoplasm. In such terms, the ongoing dimensions of brain involvement by a malignant glioma testify to a regional involvement as significant modulator in the evolutionary redefinition of therapeutic efforts to control recurrence of the local and diffuse components of injury to tumor cells.

Evolution

The incremental evolution of the proliferative indices of involvement incorporates the remodulation of systems for persistence of the neoplastic lesion. Energy metabolism is aberrantly geared towards aerobic glycolysis in most human cancers and ketogenic or low-glycemic diets have been proposed as an anti-neoplastic strategy in glioma patients [4]. In such terms, the significance of delivery of radiotherapy and of additional immunotherapy measures incorporate the outline definition of a series of radiobiologic parameters as determined within systems of strictly regional definition. Current efforts are focused on the development of novel treatment approaches, particularly on molecular targeted agents and immunotherapy [5]. It is further to regional characterization that both strictly local and strictly diffuse dimensions of glioma growth implicate the proliferative activity as injury to cellular components of the lesion and entail an additional parametric redefinition of neoplastic pathobiology. CNS development, organization and function share common features with glioma progression and malignant behaviour: these include mechanisms of proliferation and migration, interactions with microenvironment and integration into multicellular networks [6].

REFORMULATION

Encompassed reformulation of the glioma biology within spheres of operative non-accession incorporate a realization of tumor growth and also incorporated infiltration as indices of inoperability that dimensionally involve strictly regional phenomena of vascularity and immune accession as redefined by a diffuse brain affliction on the one hand and of systems of parent lesion persistence. Recently, using electromagnetic fields as a targeted mode of therapy for tumors has been proposed [7]. In such terms. the overall incongruity of systems of operative manipulation is simply an outgrowth phenomenon that modulates the mechanics of tumor recurrence. The performance of parameters of loss of control of tumor mechanics incorporate the realization of persistence of tumor growth within the biologic redefinition of the pathway characterizations of simple replacement modulation that are fundamentally based on priorization of the dynamics of infiltration of normal surrounding brain tissue. High-field intraoperative MRI neuronavigated surgery provides maximal extent of glioma resection whatever the type of glioma and location, including "staged volume" surgery [8].

The realization of pathways of incongruent dimensions of infiltration is inherent characters of paramount nature in further redefinition of injury to normal tissues. Metabolomics is an analysis of endogenous and exogenous small molecules and provides functional readouts of cellular activity that constitute cancer biology and brain tumour biology [9].

PATHOBIOLOGY

A strictly regional reformulation of activities in the pathobiology of glioma parameters of persistence. hence, is systems of intrinsic performance of a phenomenon that carries the mechanics of infiltrative growth within the performance dimensions of inherent characterization of systemic persistence in the first instance. Restoring the expression of miR-218, a microRNA commonly down regulated in glioma, dramatically reduces the migration, invasion and proliferation of glioma cells; also, miR-218 regulates many genes involved in glioma cell development, including Wnt pathways that suppress glioma cell stem-like attributes [10]. The distributional tendencies for infiltration are artifact determinants in the overall outline modulation of such persistent growth of the parent lesion. The incorporation of accessory factors is simply a performance mechanics that performs system characterization of the normal brain tissues.

The realization of induced action within the sphere of operabilities is perforce dimensions of involvement of a lesion that primarily is regional and only secondarily local or infiltrative. In such terms, ongoing performance is staged within the encompassed expression of a tumor that is highly proliferative. Glioma stem cells are located in specialised niches within tumors and mechanisms include the hypoxia dependent stimulation of angiogenesis, recruitment of endothelial progenitor cells and direct transdifferentiation into endothelial cells; they also recruit and modulate functionality of various immune cells to suppress anti-timor immune responses and foster tumor-promoting inflammation [11].

INTEGRATION

The corporate integration of a system dimension is the underlying basis of a developmental incorporation of the persistent proliferation of the individual glioma cells. In such terms, the offshoot increments of vascularization of the parent lesion are inherent characters of pathobiologic predetermination. The emerging historic concept for further growth of the tumor lesion determines the specificity of a pathology that is paramount consideration of a prior tendency to infiltrate normal brain tissue.

Such a concept allows for the realization of systems of paramount regional nature in the system recharacterization of the neoplastic proliferative activity. Within schemes of intense proliferative activity, infiltration by tumor cells is parent to both persistent growth of the local primary lesion and also for its strong tendency for recurrence after operative debulking.

Recent molecular characterisation of tutor cells together with new insights into cellular diversification during development and the modelling of these processes in transgenic animals have allowed detailed understanding of gliomagenesis [12]. Glioma stem cells are believed to underlie glioma initiation, evolution, and resistance to existing modes of therapy [13].

The redefinition of such strict parametric de-control allow for systems to be primarily mechanistic in nature and that the overall characterizations of the glioma are simply attributes of replacement of cells of non-mitotic determination.

SYSTEM SCHEMES

Systems of operative delivery as offered by immunotherapy are hence the distributional mechanics as parameters of modulated outline performance as itself delivered by various radiotherapeutic modalities and as further defined by the incremental dosage performance for further infiltration of normal brain tissues.

In this regard, the outline characters of the infiltrative performance are incremental dimensions for persistence and recurrence of the parent lesion. Glioma stem cells are increasingly aggressive in recurrent tumors with malignant progression [14]. The emergence of injury is thus a character of identity within the mechanistic performance of highly proliferative tumor beds as depicted by the further redefinition of the mechanics of replacement.

CONCLUSION

The mechanistic model for performance of strictly regional characterization of a glioma lesion is deterministic performance of injury that is reproduced by a highly proliferative pathology as schematically incorporated with strict systems for reproduction. Schemes of such nature are inherently superior to the outline dynamics of a primarily local performance of a given tumor lesion in terms that persistent and recurrence pathology offer. In such terms, the ongoing dynamics of incorporation call into operation a field performance that incorporates dimensions of inclusion within the simple infiltrative behaviour as denoted by the emergence of pathways of highly proliferative activity and of incongruent re-characterization of such intense proliferation.

The emergence of parameters for such incorporation subserve the additional predetermination set by normal brain tissues including the revascularization of systems of operative infiltration as strictly mechanistic pathways of repeated reduplication of cell division and inclusion within the parent regional lesion.

REFERENCES

[1] Chen R, Smith-Cohn M, Cohen AL, Colman H "Glioma subclassifications and their clinical significance" *Neurotherapeutics* 2017;14(2):284-297.

[2] Peng X, Liu C, Wu M "New insights into long noncoding RNAs and their roles in glioma" *Mol Cancer* 2011;17(1):61.

[3] Colquhoun A "Cell biology—metabolic crosstalk in glioma" Int J Biochem *Cell Biol* 2017;89:171-181.

[4] Winter SF, Loebel F, Dietrich J "Role of ketogenic metabolic therapy in malignant glioma: a systematic review" *Crit Rev Oncol Hematol* 2017;112:41-58.

[5] Continuum (Minneap Minn) 2017;23(6 Neuro-oncology):1548-1563.

[6] Jung E, Alfonso J, Osswald M, Monyer H, Wick W, Winkler F "Emerging intersections between neuroscience and glioma biology" *Nat Neurosci* 2000;22(12):1951-1960.

[7] Xu W, Sun J, Le Y, Chen J, Lu X, Yao X "Effect of pushed millisecond current magnetic field on the proliferation of C6 rat glioma cells" *Electromagnet Biol Med* 2010;185:197.

[8] Leroy HA, Delmaire C, Le Rhun E, Drumez E, Lejeune JP, Reyns N "High-field intraoperative MRI and glioma surgery: results after the first 100 consecutive patients" *Acta Neurochir* (Wein):2019; 61(7):1467-1474.

[9] Pandey R, Catflisch L, Lodi A, Brenner AJ, Tiziani S "Metabolomic signature of brain cancer" *Mol Carcinog* 2017;56(11):2355-2371/

[10] Tu Y, Gao X, Li G, Fu H, Cui D, Liu H et al. "MicroRNA-218 inhibits glioma invasion, migration, proliferation, and cancer stem-like cell self-renewal by targeting the polycomb group gene Bmi1" *Caner Res* 2013;73(19):6046-55.

[11] Filatova A, Acker T, Garvalov BK "The cancer stem cell niche(s): the crosstalk between glioma stem cells and their microenvironment" *Biochim Biophys Acta* 2013;1830(2)"2496-508.

[12] Westphal M, Lamszus K "The neurobiology of gliomas: from cell biology to the development of therapeutic approaches" *Nat Rev Neurosci* 2011;12(9):495-508.

[13] Suva ML, Tirosh I "The glioma cell model in the era of single-cell genomics" *Cancer Cell* 2020; 37(5):630-636.

[14] Huang Q, Zhang QB, Dong J, Wu YY, Shen YT, Zhao YD et al. "Glioma stem cells are more aggressive in recurrent tutors with malignant progression than in the primary tutor, and both can be maintained long-term in vitro" *BMC Cancer* 2008;8:304.

Chapter 20

FORMULATION OF AN INTEGRAL ANTITUMOR IMMUNE RESPONSE

ABSTRACT

Compound processes of integration of the antitumor immune response necessitates a realized dimension of process definition, on the one hand, and of further binding mechanics that implicate a broadened mechanics of binding of antibody with the targeted antigens. The evolutionary exposure of antigens is itself such a process of inherent antigenicity of whole clones and subclones of tumor cells derived from the accompanying activation of the integral immune system response. Participating factors in a network of integral dimensions are implicated within a tumor microenvironment that modulates both tumor cell biology and the immune response.

INTRODUCTION

The question of availability of monoclonal antibodies concerns the development of passively acquired or post-vaccination titers within the encompassed relative phenomenon of inducible immunity to a potentially wide range of antigen epitopes expressed on the surface membrane of tumor cells. Effectiveness of immunotherapy depends on the baseline immune response and on unleashing of pre-existing immunity [1]. In such terms, ongoing efforts to enhance specificity of antigenicity require the creation of multi-variable antigen epitopes as directive phenomenon in enhanced antitumor immune response. A unifying conceptual framework of cancer immunoeding integrates the immune system's dual host-protective and tumor-enhancing roles [2]. The intestinal micro-biome integrates environmental inputs such as diet with genetic and immune signals [3]. It is further to such considerations that the evolving dynamics of controlled specific immunity necessitates the evolution of the immune response built on variable epitope definition within heterogeneous tumor cells within the same tumor or between different tumors of different histology.

Intervention

The description of interventional efforts in generation of long-sustained antitumor immune responses requires a redefinition of inadequate immune participation in tumor cell reactivity. There has been a shift from a tumor cell-centered view of cancer development to a concept of a complex tumor ecosystem supporting tumor growth and spread [4]. In such terms, the emergence of derivative dimensions require a consideration also of differentiation antigens expressed on normal cells in a ubiquitous manner. An effective therapeutic strategy requires coordinate activation of tumor-specific immunity as well as increased accessibility of melanoma cells in primary lesions and distal metastases [5]. The system profile dimensions of the immune response require a re-characterization profile as a begetting phenomenon of supportive immune response within a setting of diagnostic efforts to identify the micrometastases or blood borne metastatic clusters. It is indeed necessary to consider also the potentiality of antibody reactivity of tumor cells within substantial improvement profiles of monoclonal antibodies that are especially administered and sustained.

HETEROGENEITY

Given the heterogeneity of tumor antigen presentation, the promotion profiles of tumor cell antigenicity allow for a system supported spectrum for the immune response. Tumor-infiltrating immune cells play a significant role in the promotion or inhibition of tumor growth, including infiltrating B lymphocytes [6]. In such terms the further evolution of antigenicity has been promoted by the use hybridoma plasma cell populations within systems for further enhanced derivation of the immune response. The immune infiltration composition changes at each tutor stage and particular cells have a major impact on survival: densities of T follicular helper cells and innate cells increase, whereas most T cell densities decrease, with tumor progression [7].

It is the institution of system biology profiles in the binding of tumor antigen to surface membrane antibody molecules as receptors that would further promote a sustained immune response. It is the system profiles that require the insertion of binding phenomena that indicate the continued sustained emergence of antigenicity as dynamics of an immune response borne out by reactivation of B lymphocytes, macrophages and Natural Killer cells.

BINDING MECHANICS

Binding dynamics appear to be a mechanics of contact dimensions within the phenomenon of interaction of various molecules aided by the T cell help promotion of the antibody response to tumor antigens. Also the processes involved in antigen expression present a realization that goes beyond sequestration from the immune system. Interferon signaling in cancer cells and immune cells oppose each other to establish a regulatory relationship that limits both adaptive and innate immune killing [8].

Emergence of Antigens

In such terms, the ongoing emergence of specific and pan-specific antigenicity permits the creation of system profiles of the immune response that are spectrum derived from monoclonal antibodies in general. Tissue-resident memory T cells are important in tumor immune surveillance and their close contact with tumor cells, dominant expression of checkpoint receptors and their recognition of cancer cells indicate that they are implicated in the success of immune checkpoint inhibitors in many cancers [9]. It is indeed relevant to consider the promotion of antigenicity that is specificity defined as targets of an ideal antitumor response.

It is also significant to consider the range of presented antigens on tumor cells as a further illustration of dynamics for sustained response and activation of B lymphocytes.

Pan-Immunity

The conglomerate dimensions of a pan-immune response is spectrum defined within realization phenomena as part of ongoing involvement as depicted within relative dimensions of a variable immune response, on the one hand, and of inherently evolved immune response as defined by single or multiple antigen presentation. Cellular metabolism is emerging as a key regulator of immunity that dictates myeloid cell and lymphocyte development, fate, and function [10]. In such terms, activation of effector mechanisms requires the turnover expression of presented antigens as derived from conceptual considerations of a system response. Tumor Interferon signaling regulates a multigenic resistance program to immune checkpoint blockade [11]. It is within such defined terms that antigen presentation is integral to the specific activation of defined antigens and that the immune response is primarily directed as specific activation of multi-variate clones and subclones of effector cell mechanisms. Targeting checkpoint receptors and molecules allow for therapeutic modulation of

Natural Killer cells; checkpoint events frequently co-opt otherwise as major mechanisms of immune escape by tumors [12].

PROMOTIONAL EFFORTS

Promotional efforts to integrate the immune response as parcel phenomenon with lymphocyte activation require the inherent process of response within the profile dynamics of response of the targeted tumor cells. In terms of overt immune response, such B cell activation necessitates the institution of a macrophage series of supportive measures that are in turn requirement based. The promotion of such phenomena requires a realization as put forward by systems of effectiveness borne out by the promotion of the antibody production mechanics.

Tumor cell-intrinsic and -extrinsic factors underlie tumor resistance to immune checkpoint blockers, and targeting these factors in combination with immune checkpoint blockers points to the future direction of cancer immunotherapy [13].

It is indeed necessary to consider derivative phenomena that are both specific for the targeted antigen and also spectrum-based as further ongoing immune response. The exposure of antigen on the cell membrane of tumor cells is further compounded by a process of effective immune cell activation in both defined terms and also as a broadened response to multi-varied antigenicity as presented by the tumor cells.

In early tumorigenesis Interferon-I represses tumor development via restriction of tumor cell proliferation and by inducing antitumor immune responses; it enhances antigen presentation in antigen-presenting cells and activates CD8+ T cells. In late stages of tumor progression, there is induced expression of immunosuppressive factors such as programmed cell death ligand on the surface of dendritic cells and other bone marrow cells and inhibition of antitumor immunity [14].

Promotion efforts for the realization of activation of immune cells is hence integral to antigen presentation in a broadened profile of antigenicity as derived dimension for further sustained response to targeted tumor cells.

In such terms, the overt process of sequestration of antigens from the immune system behoves dimensions for the persistent evolution of the immune response itself. It is significant to consider the profile printing of phenomena of immune response as derived dimension, as well defined by tumor cell damage and death of whole clones of such neoplastic cells.

CONCLUSION

By and large, the process of antigen exposure and presentation to the immune system is fully integral to dimensions for promotion in the process dynamics of activation of the targeting potentialities of antigen production by activated B lymphocytes as supported by a whole series of supporting phenomena.

The T cell support in antibody targeting requires the cooperative mechanisms of a whole series of processes of antigen ingestion by macrophages, and T cell support. Circulation of lymphocytes within the encompassed processes of exposure of B lymphocytes requires the evolving B cell site promotion within lymphoid follicles within lymph nodes, spleen and the gastrointestinal tract as evidenced by mounting dynamics of cell antigenicity.

Participation of such immune response as terms of target motivation within the tumor lesion requires dimensions of cooperation as defined by system profiles of congruent support. The potentiality for activation of such integral immune response necessitates a broadened concept of the immune response as defined pan-specificity within an inherently heterogeneous tumor cell population. Indeed, strict clonality of response and of targeting allows for evolutionary considerations as promoted by a process of antigen presentation that is primarily spectrum-defined in terms of antigen expression and B lymphocyte activation mechanics. Binding promotion consists of semi-specific exposure processes of antigens and of the activation of an integral immune response.

REFERENCES

[1] Galon J, Bruni D "Approaches to treat immune hot, altered and cold tutors with combination immunotherapies" *Nat Rev Drug Discov* 2019;18(3): 197-218.

[2] Schreiber RD, Old LJ, Smyth MJ "Cancer immunoediting: integrating immunity's roles in cancer suppression and promotion" *Science* 2011; 331(6024):1565-70.

[3] Thaiss CA, Zmora N, Levy M, Elinav E "The micro biome and innate immunity" *Nature* 2016;535(7610):65-74.

[4] Pitt JM, Marabelle A, Eggermont A, Soria JC, Kroemer G, Zitvogel L "Targeting the tumor microenvironment: removing obstruction to anticancer immune responses and immunotherapy" *Ann Oncol* 2016;27(8):1482-92.

[5] Marzagalli M, Ebelt ND, Manuel ER "Unraveling the crosstalk between melanoma and immune cells in the tutor microenvironment" *Semin Cancer Biol* 2019;59:236-250.

[6] Wang SS, Liu W, Ly D, Xu H, Qu L, Zhang L "Tumor-infiltrating B cells: their role and application n anti-tumor immunity in lung cancer" *Cell Mol Immunol* 2019;16(1):6-18.

[7] Bindea G, Mlecnik B, Tosolini M, Kirilovsky A, Waldner M, Obenauf AC et al. "Spatiotemporal dynamics of intratumoral immune cells reveal the immune landscape in human cancer" *Immunity* 2013;39(4)782-95.

[8] Bench JL, Johnson LR, Choa R, Xi Y, Qiu J, Zhou Z et al. "Opposing functions of interferon coordinate adaptive and innate immune responses to cancer immune checkpoint blockade" *Cell* 2019;178(4):933-948.

[9] Mami-Chouaib F, Blanc C, Corgnac S, Hans S, Malenica I, Granier C et al. "Resident memory T cells, critical components in tumor immunology" *J Immunother Cancer* 2018;6(1):87.

[10] Palazon A, Goldrath AW, Nizet V, Johnson RS "HIF transcription factors, inflammation, and immunity" *Immunity* 2014;41(4):618-28.

[11] Bench JL, Johnson LR, Choa R, Xu Y, Qiu J, Xhou Z et al. “Opposing functions of Interferon coordinate adaptive and innate immune responses to cancer immune checkpoint blockade” *Cell* 2016;167(6):1540-1554.

[12] Nayoung K, Hun SK “Targeting checkpoint receptors and molecules for therapeutic modulation of Natural Killer cells” *Front Immune* 2918;9:2041.

[13] Huang Q, Lei Y, Li X, Guo F, Liu M “A highlight of the mechanisms of immune checkpoint blocker resistance” *Front Cell Dev Biol* 2020;8:580140.

[14] Zhou L, Zhang Y, Wang Y, Zhang M, Sun W, Dai T et al. “A dual role of Type I Interferons in antitumor immunity” *Adv Biosyst* 2020;4(11):e1900237.

Chapter 21

Systems of Weak Immunogenicity as Originators of Early Spread and of Incremental Tumor Cell Growth and Proliferation

Abstract

Dimensions of the dynamic increments in tumor evolution indicate the inherent nature of the tumor cells as derivative biology of a weak immunogenicity and as further dominated by the acquisition of early metastatic spread potential as carcinogenesis progresses. It is in terms of incremental growth and spread of the neoplastic cells that the proliferation of such cells proves an originator of the performance profiles of network operability within systems of pronounced amplification of the weak immunogenicity as exhibited by the neoplastic cells.

Introduction

The combination of various immunotherapeutic agents, in particular the bolus injection modules of administration of interleukin 2, has shown a therapeutic effect in a small population of metastatic renal cell carcinoma patients and patients with melanoma. As such, the realization of therapeutic effect is beset by the development of significant toxicity in these patients. Therefore, there have been several attempts at combination therapy, particularly the combination of interferon alpha with interleukin 2 with the aim of achieving synergistic action against the tumors.

The modulatory effects of a direct anti-proliferative action of interferon alpha on tumor cells are a significant facet in the overall anti-tumor strategy in melanoma and renal cell carcinoma patients. These two types of tumors, particularly melanoma, serve as important models in the outline attempts at formulating strategies against most other solid-type tumors. It is the realization of both direct and indirect actions against tumor cells that attempts at combinatory immunotherapy have been formulated for future strategy.

The number of disseminated tumor cells and their karyotypic abnormalities are similar for small and large tumors in patients and mouse models [1]. In carcinoma progression, epithelial to mesenchymal transition plays a crucial role in early steps of metastasis when cells lose cell to cell-contacts [2].

Systems Of Toxicity

The overall systems of toxicity are significant in terms of such organ systems as hepatotoxicity that often prove a limiting effect in the administration of immunotherapeutic agents to tumor patients. The systems of continuous rather than bolus administration modules may prove advantageous in terms of limiting toxicity modules, but such attempts are further compromised in terms of lack of efficacy of anti-tumor effect in the vast majority of patients with metastatic melanoma or metastatic renal cell carcinoma.

Tumor Growth and Proliferation

In terms of realization in the control of tumor cell growth and proliferation, it is significant to consider the terms of reference in models of cancer cell biology. Natural killer cells contribute to the first line of defence against tumor growth and metastasis spread [3]. Combination immunotherapy to such agents as chemotherapy, and in the strategic attempts of anti-tumor effect, is significant within focused attack against multiple biologic facets of tumor cell proliferation and growth and also especially in the control of metastatic biology. Incorporating immune-molecular targets into combination as well as refining the standard chemotherapy might unlock the future of triple-negative breast cancer [4].

Understanding how selective pressure from chemotherapy directs the evolution of urothelial carcinoma and shapes, its clonal architecture is crucial [5].

It is particularly significant to view the complex scenario of tumor cell biology as systems of inter-related events that potentiate each other, with the overall aim at restricting metastatic potential of neoplastic cells. Combining cancer vaccine and checkpoint blockade for treating HPV-related cancer is a promising approach [6].

Network Operabilities

The increments in tumor cell growth, proliferation and spread are paramount considerations as the tumor progresses clinically and pathophysiologically. The identification of molecular markers could early predict the metastatic potential of tumors such as thyroid cancer [7]. The performance strategies of tumor effects are a complex phenomenon in terms of the evolutionary potentials of neoplastic cells in general. Epithelial-mesenchymal transition is a crucial step in cancer progression and plays a key role in tumor metastasis [8]. A network approach is based on the realization of complex interactions that emphasize, in particular, the antigen presentation by professional cells such as dendritic cells. This formulation approach is further significant within scopes of multi-organ spread of neoplasms in general. It is in terms of such network operabilities that the overall clinical dimensions of tumor spread further illustrate the dynamics of growth and spread of tumor cells.

Inclusive phenomena in the performance, in particular, of growth of neoplastic cells, are the weak immunogenicity of tumor cells. The multi-step reprogramming process resulting in a phenotype switch from an epithelial to a mesenchymal cellular state has been closely related to the acquisition of stem cell-like attributes in tumors [9]. Laminin-5 with transforming growth factor-beta1 induces epithelial to mesenchymal transition in hepatocellular carcinoma [10]. The exposure of antigenic epitopes is a central consideration in the performance attempts with the realization of antigen-presenting cells infiltrating the tumor itself. In such terms, interleukin 2 effects are potentiation as expansion performance on such infiltrating tumor lymphocytes. The emergence of such a concept is the complexities of performance of antigen presentation by dendritic cells.

Dimensions of Epitope Biology

Overall dimensions in the antigen epitope biology are emphasized as central to such tumors as metastatic melanoma. The incremental functionalities of realization are emphasized by the recognition of early phase dynamics as terms of self-potentiating factors in performance agency against the tumor in question. Hence, the importance of early phase tumor cell growth and proliferation is underlined by the essential need to prevent self-potentiation of the tumor biology dynamics. Transforming growth factor-beta induces epithelial-mesenchymal transition in hepatocellular carcinoma and probably also changes in tumor cell plasticity [11].

It is significant to view the essential evolutionary history of a tumor lesion as primarily self-potentiating, even as the neoplastic cells initiate spread very early in the course of growth and proliferation. Tumor-Associated macrophages promote cancer stem cell-like properties via transforming growth factor-beta1-induced epithelial-mesenchymal transition in hepatocellular carcinoma [12].

Weak Immunogenicity and Metastases

Profile systems of antigenicity are inherent within the systems of carcinogenicity as projected by the increments of progression of the metastatic potential. In real terms, the ability of neoplastic cells to spread early in the course of carcinogenesis is highly significant, and is in fact suggestive of an intrinsic potentiality of the tumorigenesis that is inherent to the metastatic potential of a given tumor lesion. The synergistic interactions exist between CD44 and transforming growth factor-Beta1 in epithelial mesenchymal transition induction and of cancer stem cell properties through the AKT/GSK-3Beta/Beta-catenin pathway in hepatocellular carcinoma cells [13]. In such terms, it appears significant to consider antigenicity within the central phenomenon of early spread of the tumor cells. Such a concept would lead to a realization of growth and proliferation as epiphenomena of such early metastatic capability and operability of the neoplastic cells, in focused terms.

Early Spread Potential

Such a concept therefore reverts the question of early spread as an originator of escalating incremental phenomena of the growth and spread of the tumor cells, inherently operating a poor immunogenicity phenomenon. In such terms, therefore, the weak immunogenicity of tumor cells, both in general and specific terms, operates as a fundamental instigator in the incremental growth and proliferation of the neoplastic cells.

Conclusion

Systems of profile performance are inherent models of incremental growth and proliferation of tumor cells very early in the acquisition of metastatic spread potential of these cells. It is in terms of overall performance that the increments of tumor spread are translated in as increments of growth and spread of tumor cells as group biology of lesion pathophysiology. The dynamics of incremental growth and proliferation are central to metastatic potential that directly implicates weak immunogenicity of the tumor cells.

References

[1] Husemann Y, Geigl JB, Schubert F, Musiani P, Meyer M, Burghart E et al. "Systemic spread is an early step in breast cancer" *Cancer Cell* 2008; 13(1):58-68.

[2] Giannelli G, Koudelkova P, Dituri F, Mikulits W "Role of epithelial to mesenchymal transition in hepatocellular carcinoma" *J Hepatic* 2016;65(4):798-808.

[3] Pende D, Falco M, Vitale M, Cantoni C, Vitale C, Munari E et al. "Killer Ig-like receptors (KIRs): their role in NK cell modulation and developments leading to their clinical exploitation" *Front Immune* 2019;10:1179.

[4] Park JH, Ahn JH, Kim SB "How shall we treat early triple-negative breast cancer (TNBC): from the current standard to upcoming immune-molecular strategies" *ESMO Open* 2018;3 (Suppl 1): e000357.

[5] Faltas BM, Prandi D, Tarawa ST, Molina AM, Nanus DM, Sternberg C et al. "Clonal evolution of chemotherapy-resistant urothelial carcinoma" *Nat Genet* 2016;48(12):1490-1499.

[6] Shibata T, Lieblong BJ, Sasagawa T, Nakagawa M "The promise of combining cancer vaccine and checkpoint blockade for treating HPV-related cancer" *Cancer Treat Rev* 2019;78-8.

[7] Gugnoni M, Sancisi V, Gandolfi G, Manzotti G, Ragazzi M, Giordano D et al. "Cadherin-6 promotes EMT and cancer metastasis by restraining autophagy" *Oncogene* 2017;36(5):667-677.

[8] Da C, Wu K, Yue C, Bai P, Wang R, Wang G et al. "N-cadherin promotes thyroid tumorigenesis through modulating major signaling pathways" *Oncotarget* 2017;8(9):e75489.

[9] Jayachandran A, Dhungel B, Steel JC "Epithelial-to-mesenchymal plasticity of cancer stem cells: therapeutic targets in hepatocellular carcinoma" *J Hematol Oncol* 2016;9(1):74.

[10] Giannelli G, Bergamini C, Fransvea E, Sgarra C, Intonaci S "Laminin-5 with transforming growth factor-beta1 induces epithelial to mesenchymal transition in hepatocellular carcinoma" *Gastroenterology* 2005;129(5):1375-83.

[11] Fan QM, Jing YY, Yu GF, Kou XR, Ye F, Gao L et al. "Tumor-associated macrophages promote cancer stem cell-like properties via transforming growth factor-beta1-induced epithelial-mesenchymal transition in hepatocellular carcinoma" *Cancer Lett* 2014;352(2):160-8.

[12] Malfettone A, Soukupova J, Bertran E, Crosas-Molist E, Lastra R, Fernando J et al. "Transforming growth factor-beta-induced plasticity causes a migratory stemless phenotype in hepatocellular carcinoma" *Cancer Lett* 2017;392-39-50.

[13] Park NR, Cha JH, Jang JW, Bae SH, Jang B, Kim JH et al. "Synergistic effects of CD44 and TGF-beta1 through AKT/GSK-3beta/beta-catenin singling during epithelial-mesenchymal transition in liver cancer cells" *Biochem Biophys Res Commun* 2016;477(4):568-574.

About the Author

Lawrence M. Agius

The author of this monograph is a retired senior lecturer and consultant histopathologist and neuropathologist. He has been a visiting professor in neuropathology at Ohio State University and senior visiting fellow at the Neurology Institute in Queen's Square in London UK. He has practiced as consultant for over 20 years at Mater Dei and has delivered many lectures and tutorials to graduate and postgraduate students. He has been for many years Head of the section of histopathology and clinical cytology He is the author of over 200 published articles and 4 books.

INDEX

A

B

C

D

G

T